Understanding Common Disorders in Reproductive Endocrinology

Understanding Common Disorders in Reproductive Endocrinology

Edited by

Michael M. Dooley
Mark P. Brincat

JOHN WILEY & SONS
Chichester · New York · Brisbane · Toronto · Singapore

Baffins Lane, Chichester,
West Sussex PO19 1UD, England
Telephone: National, Chichester (0243) 779777
International, +44 243 779777

Other Wiley Editorial Offices

John Wiley & Sons, Inc., 605 Third Avenue,
New York, NY 10158–0012, USA

Jacaranda Wiley Ltd, 33 Park Road, Milton,
Queensland 4064, Australia

John Wiley & Sons (Canada) Ltd, 22 Worcester Road,
Rexdale, Ontario M9W 1L1, Canada

John Wiley & Sons (SEA) Pte Ltd, 37 Jalan Pemimpin #05–04,
Block B, Union Industrial Building, Singapore 2057

Library of Congress Cataloging-in-Publication Data

Understanding common disorders in reproductive endocrinology / edited
by Michael M. Dooley and Mark P. Brincat.
p. cm.
Includes bibliographical references and index.
ISBN 0 471 94151 4
Endocrine gynecology. I. Dooley, Michael M. II. Brincat,
Mark P.
[DNLM: 1. Reproduction—physiology. 2. Infertility—
physiopathology. 3. Menstruation Disorders—physiopathology.
4. Contraceptive Agents, Female. WP 550 U55 1994]
RG159.U53 1994
618.1—dc20
DNLM/DLC
for Library of Congress 93-20863
CIP

British Library Cataloguing in Publication Data

A catalogue record for this book is available from the British Library

ISBN 0 471 94151 4

Typeset by Inforum, Rowlands Castle, Hants
Printed and bound in Great Britain by Biddles Ltd, Guildford

Contents

Contributors

Ricardo H. Asch MD
University of California, Irvine, California 92717, USA

Mark P. Brincat MRCS, LRCP, PhD(Lond), MRCOG
Department of Obstetrics and Gynaecology, St Luke's Hospital Medical School, Malta

Michael Chapman MD, MRCOG
Academic Division of Obstetrics and Gynaecology, United Medical and Dental Schools, Guy's Hospital Campus, London Bridge, London SE1 9RT, UK

D. C. Costigan FRCPI, FRCP(C)
Department of Paediatric Endocrinology, Our Lady's Hospital for Sick Children, Crumlin, Dublin, Ireland

P.G. Crosignani MD
Department of Obstetrics and Gynaecology, University of Milan, Via Commenda 12, 20122 Milan, Italy

Michael M. Dooley MMs(NUI), MRCOG
Department of Obstetrics and Gynaecology, West Dorset Hospital, Damers Road, Dorchester DT1 2JY, UK

Marc Formosa MD, MRCOG
Department of Obstetrics and Gynaecology, St Luke's Hospital Medical School, Malta

Mary L. Forsling PhD
Department of Obstetrics and Gynaecology, United Medical and Dental Schools, St Thomas' Hospital Campus, Lambeth Palace Road, London SE1 7EH, UK

Jane L. Frederick MD
University of California, Irvine, California 92717, USA

Colm O'Herlihy MD, FRCPI, FRCOG, FRACOG
Department of Obstetrics and Gynaecology, University College Dublin, National Maternity Hospital, Holles Street, Dublin 2, Ireland

Neil Pickering
Centre for the Study of Philosophy and Health Care, University College Swansea, Singleton Park, Swansea SA2 8PP, UK

Adam Rodin BSc, MRCOG
Department of Obstetrics and Gynaecology, United Medical and Dental Schools, Guy's Hospital Campus, London Bridge, London SE1 9RT, UK

C. La Vecchia
Mario Negri Institute, Milan, Italy

Introduction

Due to the fact that the understanding of female reproductive endocrinology is developing at a rapid rate, the knowledge of many general clinicians is left behind. However, many clinical problems are met, on a daily basis, in the general surgery and it is the purpose of this book to help practising clinicians in their day-to-day work.

We have been very fortunate in obtaining contributions from clinicians throughout the world with up-to-date knowledge of the subject, often based on their personal research.

Medical students often find reproductive endocrinology a problem. We hope that the chapters in this book will enhance their appreciation and understanding of this most fascinating area of medicine.

We would like to thank all those who have helped in the production of this book, especially the staff of John Wiley for their support and patience based on years of specialised experience in medical publishing.

1

The Anatomy of the Reproductive Tract and the Physiology of the Menstrual Cycle

Mary L. Forsling
United Medical and Dental Schools,
St Thomas' Hospital Campus, London, UK

Great genetic diversity in a population results from sexual reproduction, the essential feature of which is that an individual transmits only half its chromosomes to the next generation, either via the male gamete, the sperm, or via the female gamete, the ovum. The gametes are formed from germ cells by reduction division, known as meiosis, when the chromosome number is halved and the composition of each chromosome modified as a result of chromosomal exchange. When the gametes come together on fertilisation a zygote is formed. The gametes are produced in the gonads, which additionally elaborate hormones that shape not only the anatomy and physiology of the individual, but also behaviour and aspects of social function.

The uterus and menses were recognised several millenia before the ovary was identified. The Sumerian birth goddess Nintu was shaped like a uterus and the Egyptian hieroglyph *Ankh* depicted on the birth goddess Taurt resembles a uterus. Discovery of the ovary is attributed to Herophilus of Chalcedon, an anatomist of the Alexandrian school of the fourth century. In classical literature the term female testicle was used, so that the anatomical analogy was recognised, although its function was unknown. According to Aristotle (384–322 BC) the seed produced in the male ducts developed in the soil of the menstrual coagulation of the female. The study of the gamete may be considered to have been initiated in 1647 when Leeuwehoek and Ham first described human sperm seen under the microscope. Some 26 years earlier Harvey had proposed that an egg was the common origin of all

Understanding Common Disorders in Reproductive Endocrinology. Edited by M.M. Dooley and M.P. Brincat.

animals, but it was not until 1822 that von Bauer published his description of its formation. The possibility that the gonads also produced hormones arose from the experiments of Berthold, who in 1849 showed that transplantation of a cock's testes into a capon induced normal development of the comb in the castrated animal. Ovarian oestrogens were isolated and purified between 1919 and 1930, followed by purification of progesterone. One further important milestone was the suggestion of Moore and Price in 1932 that gonadal steroid hormones could influence the release of gonadotrophins.

ANATOMY AND EMBRYOLOGY OF THE FEMALE REPRODUCTIVE SYSTEM

The gonads in the human begin to develop around the fifth week of gestation. They are derived from two distinct tissues: somatic and mesenchymal tissues, which form the matrix of the gonad; and the primordial germ cells which migrate into the matrix and form the gametes. The early development proceeds identically in both sexes. At the end of this indifferent phase of development the urogenital tract comprises two components. These are the dual duct systems (the Wolffian and the Müllerian), consisting of the urogenital sinus and tubules which differentiate to form the external genitalia. Sexual differentiation must be actively diverted along the male line. Thus in the female, in the absence of testicular secretions, the Müllerian ducts develop and differentiate into female reproductive organs, while the Wolffian ducts degenerate (Figure 1).

The reproductive organs of the female (Figure 2) comprise the vagina, the uterus, the uterine tubes and the ovaries. The vagina is a muscular tube about 10–15 cm long which passes from the vulva upwards and backwards between the bladder and the rectum. The walls comprise smooth muscle and fibroelastic tissue lined with a mucous membrane of stratified squamous epithelium thrown into transverse folds (rugae). The vaginal wall is capable of constriction and enormous dilation. At its superior end the vagina is continuous with the cervix—the lower part of the uterus. Recesses known as the anterior, posterior and lateral fornices are formed around the projecting cervix. The lining of the vagina does not contain any glandular cells, but is moistened by secretions of the cervix and the glands of the vestibule. The mucus secreted by the cervix is acidified to a pH between 4 and 6 by the action of vaginal bacteria, mainly lactobacilli acting on glycogen from the cells of the vaginal epithelium. The acidic environment helps to safeguard the pelvic organs from infection as it inhibits the growth of micro-organisms. Over the course of the menstrual cycle there are regular changes in the cells of the vaginal lining, so that vaginal smears can indicate the time

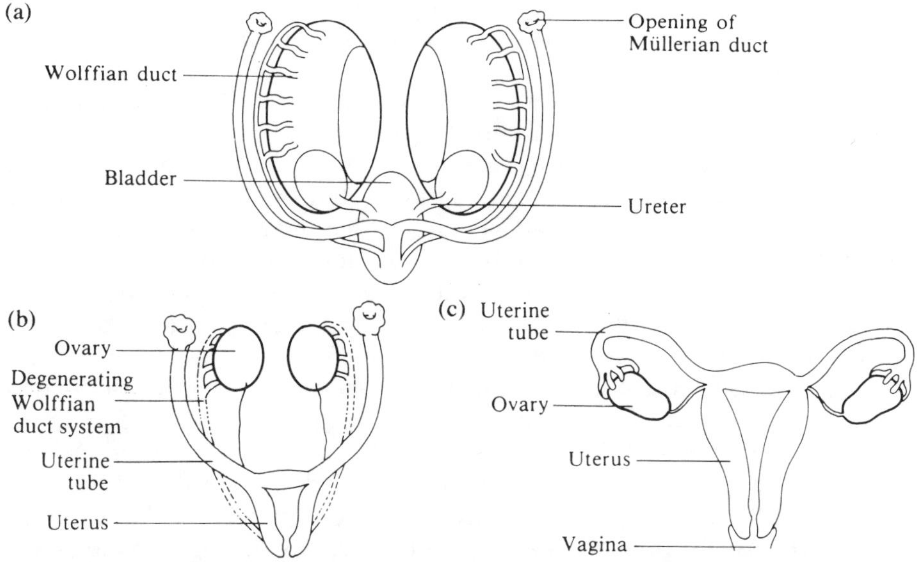

Figure 1 Development of the female reproductive system from structures originally common to male and female. (a) Duct systems. (b) Developing female structures. (c) Mature female reproductive tract. Reproduced from Stanier, M.W. and Forsling, M.L. (1989). *Physiological Processes: An Introduction to Mammalian Physiology*, by permission of McGraw Hill

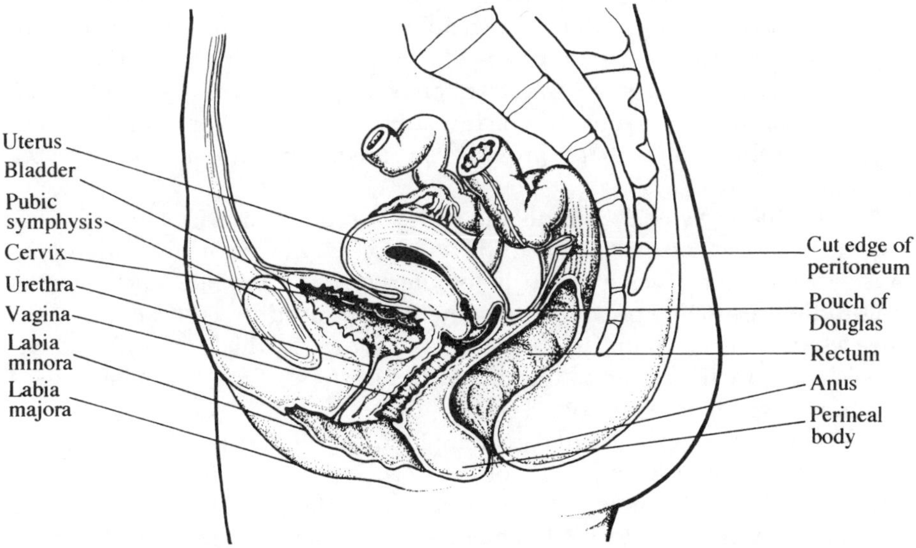

Figure 2 The normal female pelvis in sagittal section. Reproduced by permission of R.W. Taylor

of ovulation. More importantly, cervical smears are taken in the Pap test—a cytological examination originated by George Paponicolacus as a screening test for cervical cancer.

The uterus is pear-shaped and in the non-pregnant state the muscular walls are very thick, so that it is only 7.5 cm long and 5 cm across its widest part. In pregnancy of course the walls expand to hold not only a 3–4 kg infant but also the fetal fluids. Although the uterus is firmly anchored and supported in the pelvic cavity above the bladder and in front of the rectum, its position varies depending on the distension of the bladder and rectum. There are three layers to the uterine wall, the outer being a peritoneal covering that is continuous with the peritoneum of the supporting broad ligaments. The middle layer or myometrium comprises bundles of smooth muscle fibres embedded in connective tissue and forming three ill-defined interlaced layers: circular, longitudinal and spiral. The interlaced arrangement is important after childbirth as the contracting muscle compresses the blood vessels, preventing haemorrhage. The third layer of the uterus—the lining or endometrium—is a very vascular mucous membrane. Its stroma of connective tissue supports tubular epithelial glands opening into the lumen of the uterus. As with the lining of the other regions of the reproductive tract, the endometrium undergoes distinct changes over the course of the menstrual cycle.

Extending laterally from the uterus, between the layers of the broad ligaments, are the Fallopian tubes, each about 10 cm long. They do not form a completely continuous conduit from the ovaries to the uterus, but end in a funnel-shaped opening—the infundibulum—surrounded by a fringe of finger-like processes—the fimbriae—the largest of which may touch the ovary. When an ovum is released from an ovary it must cross a small gap to the Fallopian tube. A problem which results from the Fallopian tube opening into the abdomen is that it provides a route for infection to spread to the peritoneal cavity.

As with the body of the uterus the Fallopian tube comprises three layers. The muscle layer consists of a well-developed inner layer of circular smooth muscle which gets thicker towards the uterus, and a thinner outer layer of longitudinal muscle. Peristaltic movements produced by contraction of the muscles propel the ovum to the uterus—a journey which takes 3–4 days. This is aided by the action of the cilia found in some of the epithelial cells, a number of which are secretory.

The two ovaries, each about 3 cm long in the adult, lie near the lateral wall of the pelvis, connected by folds of the peritoneum with the posterior surface of the broad ligament of the uterus and attached to the uterus by a fibrous cord within the broad ligament—the ovarian ligaments. At birth the ovary contains about one million oocytes but this has fallen to 300 000 by puberty and all are lost by the menopause. A process called genetically

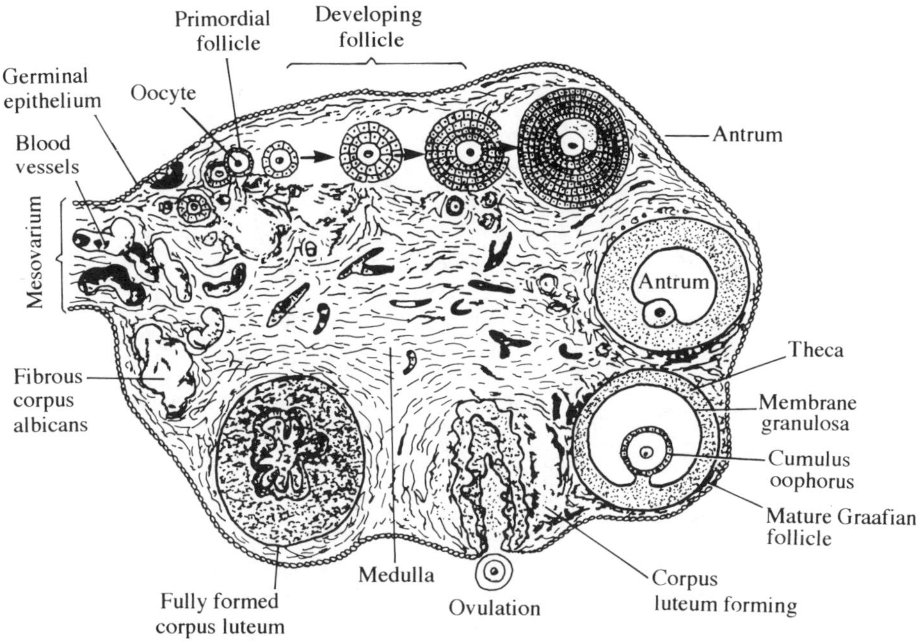

Figure 3 Diagram of the ovary showing, in clockwise progression, growth, maturation and ovulation

controlled atresia accounts for the loss of oocytes. Of the three regions of the ovary, the oocytes are contained in the outer cortex (Figure 3), which represents the greater mass of the ovary. Next there is the inner medulla, formed from the stromal cells and cells with steroid-producing characteristics, and finally the hilum, which serves as the point of entry of the nerves and blood vessels. In addition to the oocytes the follicles of the ovary have two further cellular components. These are the granulosa cells surrounding the oocytes and the theca cells which are separated by a membrane from the former.

THE OVARIAN CYCLE

Characteristic of reproduction in the female is the cyclical nature of events centred on the episodic release of oocytes on ovulation. As mentioned, in addition to the production of ova, the ovary has an endocrine function. The two main types of steroids secreted by the ovary—the oestrogens and the progestagens (Figure 4)—show an episodic release, the oestrogens dominating the pre-ovulatory phase and the gestagens the post-ovulatory phase. The

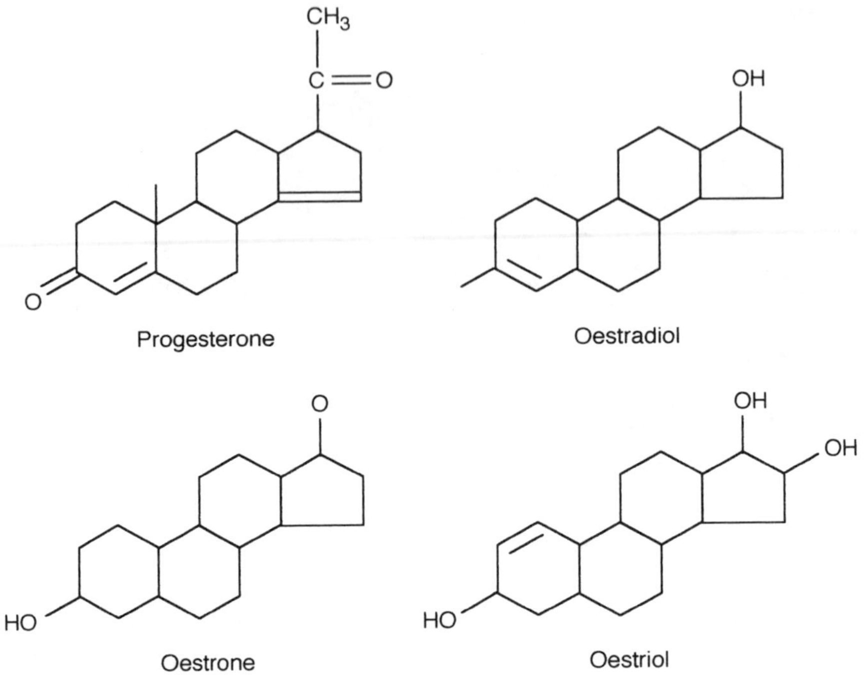

Figure 4 Structures of natural oestrogens and progesterone

cyclical release of the ovarian steroids produces cyclical events in the whole body. This is associated with the fact that the genital tract serves both as a route to transport the gametes to the site of fertilisation and as the site of implantation of the fertilised egg and its subsequent development.

At puberty a pool of developing follicles is formed and subsequently a few follicles recommence growth each cycle, increasing their size and the number of surrounding granulosa cells. These secrete glycoprotein round the oocyte, forming the zona pellucida. Gap junctions form between adjacent cells, allowing intracellular communication. Cells in the ovarian stroma become condensed around the follicle, forming the theca, which becomes vascularized. During the pre-antral phase the egg undergoes its greatest growth and the follicles develop luteinising hormone (LH) (thecal cells) and follicle-stimulating hormone (FSH) receptors, so that they are responsive to the pituitary gonadotrophins. If the gonadotrophin concentrations become too low the follicles undergo atresia, protein synthesis stops and the oocyte dies. In the presence of adequate concentrations of LH and FSH the follicle will continue to form antral or Graafian follicles—the higher the hormone concentrations the higher the number of follicles that will be saved. In the antral (follicular) phase, which lasts 8–12 days, the follicle increases in size, the theca divides into the theca externa and the theca interna, and the granulosa cells break away to form a central lumen filled with fluid, which is secreted by the granulosa cells. The egg floats in this lumen attached only by a stalk of granulosa cells and surrounded by a ring of granulosa cells, some of which allow a supply of nutrients to the egg. These are the so-called nurse cells. As these changes occur the follicle pushes up to the surface of the ovary and begins to bulge out of the ovary.

During the second phase of growth the follicles exhibit a steady increase in the synthesis of steroid hormones—androgens and oestrogens. Cholesterol is the precursor for all steroid hormones, its conversion to pregnenolone (Figure 5) being the first and common step in the formation of all major steroid hormones. This conversion is rate-limiting and therefore an important point for the hormonal regulation of steroid synthesis. It occurs in the inner mitochondrial membrane and requires NADPH (the reduced form of nicotinamide adenine dinucleotide phosphate), oxygen and cytochrome P-450. Pregnenolone is then converted to the active sex steroids. Like the precursor, all steroid hormones are poorly water-soluble and are carried in the blood in association with proteins such as albumin and special binding proteins. Being lipid-soluble steroid hormones readily enter cells to produce an effect at the cell nucleus. They may also (e.g. progesterone) affect the stability and ionic permeability of cell membranes. Present on the theca cells are LH receptors; the hormone acts at this site to stimulate the synthesis of androstenedione and testosterone, which is transferred to the granulosa cells for conversion to oestradiol. Levels of androgens in the ovarian venous blood are three times higher than those of oestrogen during the follicular phase. The granulosa cells possess receptors to FSH which act to induce aromatisation of the thecal androgens to oestrogen. The oestrogen can stimulate the formation of oestrogen receptors in the granulosa cells that act to stimulate the production of oestrogens, thus forming a positive feedback system resulting in a surge of oestrogen. Oestrogen, FSH, insulin and cortisol also act on the granulosa cells to stimulate the production of LH receptors in the outer layer of the granulosa tissue. The follicle has now entered the pre-ovulatory stage, only one follicle doing so. The rest become atretic and die. Atresia depends in part on the ratio of testosterone to oestrogen in the follicular fluids, androgens stimulating atresia, while oestrogens antagonise this effect. Thus the slightly less mature follicles producing less oestrogen will become atretic.

Regulation of function occurs at an intragonadal level. The interaction between cells within a gonad extends beyond the same cell type to include germ cell–somatic cell interaction. Local interactions probably facilitate the differing requirements of the various developmental stages of germ cells within the gonad which would not be possible by simply varying the

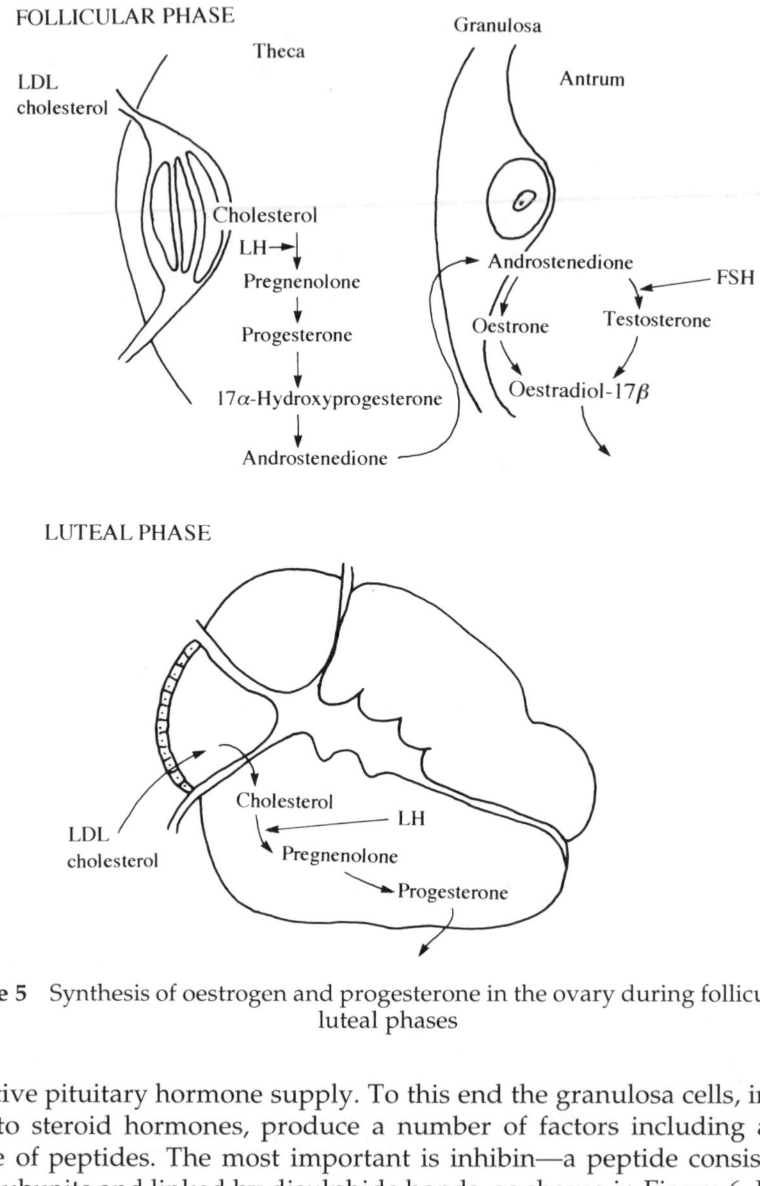

Figure 5 Synthesis of oestrogen and progesterone in the ovary during follicular and luteal phases

effective pituitary hormone supply. To this end the granulosa cells, in addition to steroid hormones, produce a number of factors including a wide range of peptides. The most important is inhibin—a peptide consisting of two subunits and linked by disulphide bonds, as shown in Figure 6. Inhibin is a specific inhibitor of FSH secretion. Synthesis of inhibin in the follicular phase is stimulated by FSH. At the time of the mid-cycle surge, inhibin is stimulated both by LH and FSH and the concentrations rise slightly. After ovulation there is a transient fall, followed by an increase in the mid-luteal phase. Another peptide, called activin, also consisting of two subunits, is

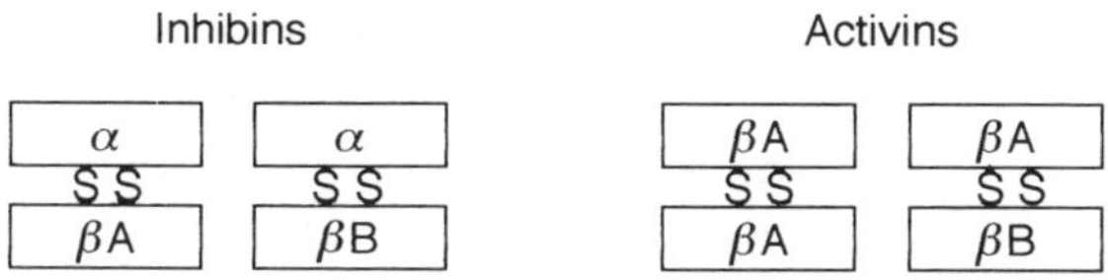

Figure 6 Structure of inhibins and activins

produced by the granulosa cells and selectively stimulates FSH release (Figure 6). A further peptide in the follicular fluid is follistatin which, like inhibin, selectively inhibits FSH release from the pituitary, but not its synthesis.

Another group of substances produced by the ovary, as in many other tissues, are growth factors. Important among these are the insulin-like growth factors (IGF-1 and IGF-2), whose production in the granulosa cells is stimulated by FSH and oestradiol. There are receptors for IGFs in both granulosa and thecal cells, so that it has both autocrine and paracrine functions. Overall they amplify the actions of the gonadotrophins, enhancing steroidogenesis, formation of LH receptors on the granulosa cells and production of inhibin. They also contribute to follicular growth and differentiation. The action appears to be additionally modified by the IGF binding proteins present in the follicular fluid, which are said to reduce IGF actions. Other growth factors include fibroblast growth factor, which is found in granulosa cells and induces proliferation of theca cells and vascularisation of the theca. Epidermal growth factor (EGF) is produced by the thecal cells and inhibits steroidogenesis and stimulates protein synthesis, including the formation of IGF. Another factor—transforming growth factor—which inhibits growth and antagonises EGF, is found in the thecal cells and follicular fluid. It interacts with FSH in low concentrations and enhances its activity, but acts to inhibit high concentrations of the hormones.

It has been found that as in other tissues there is a renin–angiotensin system, the components being formed in a 10-fold higher concentration in follicular fluid than in the peripheral circulation. They are produced under control of FSH and oestradiol by the thecal cells, the levels changing in parallel with oestradiol. They are probably involved in the formation of new blood vessels prior to ovulation and during formation of the corpus luteum. Other peptides important in controlling ovarian function include: gonadotrophin-releasing hormone (GnRH)-like peptide which in low doses stimulates and in high doses inhibits steroidogenesis; an inhibitor of luteinisation; and the placental hormones PP12, PP14, PP5 and PAA, the levels of which alter in parallel with those of oestrogen. Since the second two are inhibitors of protease, they may act to inhibit follicular rupture. The concentrations of PP14 are higher in the late luteal phase through to the early follicular phase, and as they are lower in anovulatory cycles the concentrations may be used to distinguish such cycles. There are also present many neurotransmitters, including noradrenaline, substance P, acetylcholine, vasoactive intestinal poplypeptide (VIP) and opioid peptides.

At around day 14 of the cycle the LH surge occurs, as shown in Figure 7. If this coincides with the production of granulosa LH receptors, ovulation occurs. Where there is no coincidence, the antral follicle dies. The process of ovulation has many parallels with the inflammatory process. Thus the blood flow to the follicle increases, fibroblasts within the theca proliferate and white cells invade the area. There is histamine release, a rise in plasminogen activator activity and in the production of prostaglandins E_1 and $F_{2\alpha}$. The LH surge stimulates resumption of meiosis of the oocyte, which occurs with an unequal division of the cytoplasm, the secondary oocyte possessing half the chromosomes and most of the cytoplasm. The other half is called the first polar body. The second meiotic division then commences, only to be arrested at metaphase. The process is completed at fertilisation, if it occurs, when the haploid ovum is formed together with the second polar body. It seems that the oocyte maturation inhibitor that produces the arrest of meiosis is produced by granulosa cells, higher concentrations being produced in such follicles. The levels fall as the follicles increase in size and the levels of oestradiol rise. The inhibitor acts to increase the concentrations of cyclic AMP in the cumulus cells and this then passes via gap junctions into the oocyte, where it synergises with hypoxanthine to maintain the arrested state. Meiosis is completed under the influence of the LH surge. The underlying mechanisms appear also to involve transporting hypoxanthine and the adenosine derivatives out of the egg or stimulation of a meiosis-inducing factor.

Another factor in the maturation of the follicle may be prolactin, which could contribute to the production of LH receptors. A small surge of prolactin has been noted at the same time as the LH peak. While high concentrations inhibit progesterone synthesis, low concentrations of prolactin are required for progesterone synthesis in the luteal phase. In addition to the hypothalamic inhibitory control and a possible prolactin-releasing factor which are important at specific times such as stress or lactation, prolactin release is also modulated by oestrogen. It may uncouple dopamine receptors and so block the action of dopamine and also acts on intra-pituitary factors.

Associated with the LH surge are a number of other changes that contribute to successful fertilisation. The processes of the nurse cells are withdrawn from the egg and the nurse cells lay down an extracellular matrix around the egg. The cortical granules within the eggs migrate to the periphery. After entry of a sperm they fuse with the membrane of the egg—the vitelline membrane—and release a lysosomal material that affects the zona pellucida, rendering it impermeable to other sperm.

Within 2 h of the LH surge, the hormone has stimulated progesterone production. It acts to stimulate and then inhibit the endocrine activity of the

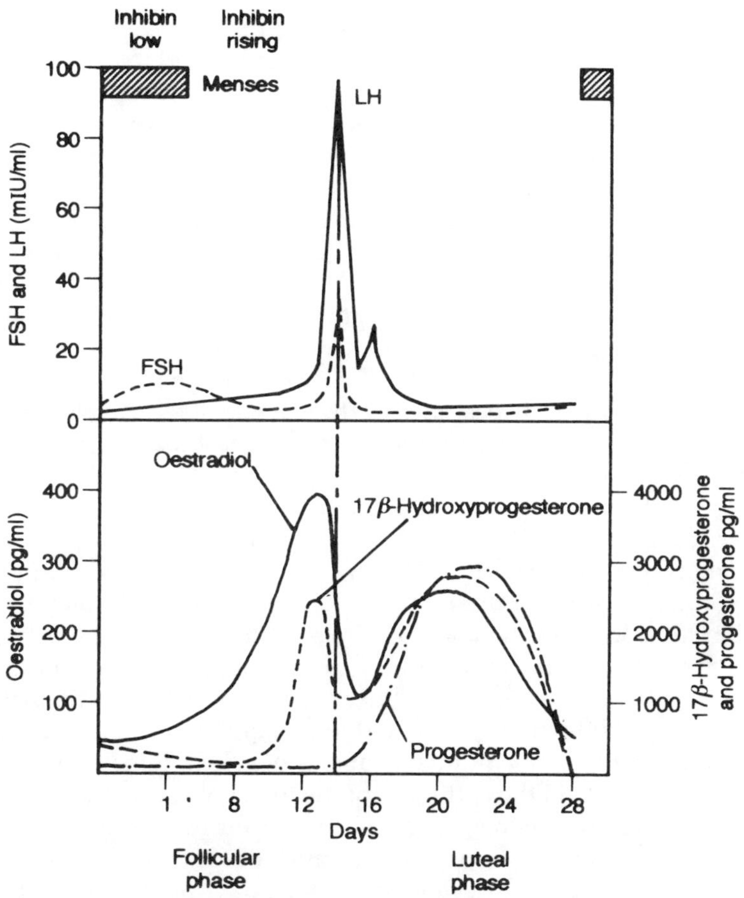

Figure 7 Changing concentrations of pituitary gonadotrophins and ovarian steroids over the menstrual cycle

thecal cells, and inhibits the aromatising activity of the granulosa cells, diverting them to the production of progesterone. Coincident with the appearance of the LH receptors are the oestrogen and the FSH receptors in the granulosa cells.

These various changes culminate in ovulation. The follicle ruptures at a point where the follicle wall becomes very thin; the stigma and the follicular fluid, which has increased greatly in volume, flows out, carrying with it the oocyte. The rupture is not due to the increased hydrostatic pressure in the follicle, but probably due to the action of plasminogen activators and of prostaglandins and histamine. Plasminogen activators are proteases that cleave plasminogen to form plasmin, which then converts the inactive pre-collagenase to collagenase. Synthesis of plasminogen activators is stimulated by gonadotrophins as well as progesterone and relaxin, so that prior to ovulation there is a large increase in the concentrations, leading to dissolution of the basal lamina and perifollicular stroma. The increased LH concentrations also enhance synthesis of prostaglandins, which act on the theca and cause it to contract.

The follicle that ruptures at the time of ovulation promptly fills with blood to form the corpus haemorrhagicum. A fibrin clot forms in the lumen of the follicle, upon which the granulosa and theca cells collapse. The clotted blood is replaced by luteal cells which hypertrophy and become spherical, with increased endoplasmis reticulum, Golgi bodies, a pigment (lutein) and lipids. The luteal cells secrete 17β-hydroxyprogesterone, progesterone and oestrogens, particularly oestradiol-17β. The role of the secreted progesterone is to prepare the endometrium to receive the fertilised egg. Endocrine support of the corpus luteum is provided by LH and, as previously mentioned, possibly prolactin. The differentiation of the follicle into the corpus luteum is under the control of LH. The effect on steroid synthesis may involve the mediation of prostaglandin E. As already indicated, in addition to steroids the corpus luteum synthesises protein and peptide hormones, including inhibin, relaxin, oxytocin and vasopressin. Relaxin is of importance during pregnancy and parturition, but may for example also act as a growth factor over the menstrual cycle. In the sheep, ovarian oxytocin stimulates prostaglandin $F_{2\alpha}$ production, which induces regression of the corpus luteum. However, the role in the human, if any, is not clear. It may serve to maintain the corpus luteum in the early part of the luteal phase and later may contribute to luteolysis. If pregnancy occurs, the corpus luteum persists and there is no further menstruation until after parturition. If there is no pregnancy the corpus luteum begins to degenerate about 4 days before the next menses. In many species it appears that luteolysis is produced by uterine prostaglandins. However, this does not appear to be the case in the human, although the involvement of local prostaglandins stimulated by oestrogen or oxytocin cannot be ruled out. An alternative possibility is that the levels are not sufficiently high to maintain the corpus luteum.

THE MENSTRUAL CYCLE

The shifting balance of hormones over the course of the ovarian cycle affects activity throughout the reproductive tract in addition to exerting a generalised effect in the body as a whole. The effects of ovarian steroids fall into the general categories: determinative, i.e. quantitative changes that are more or less irreversible; or regulatory or qualitative changes in established

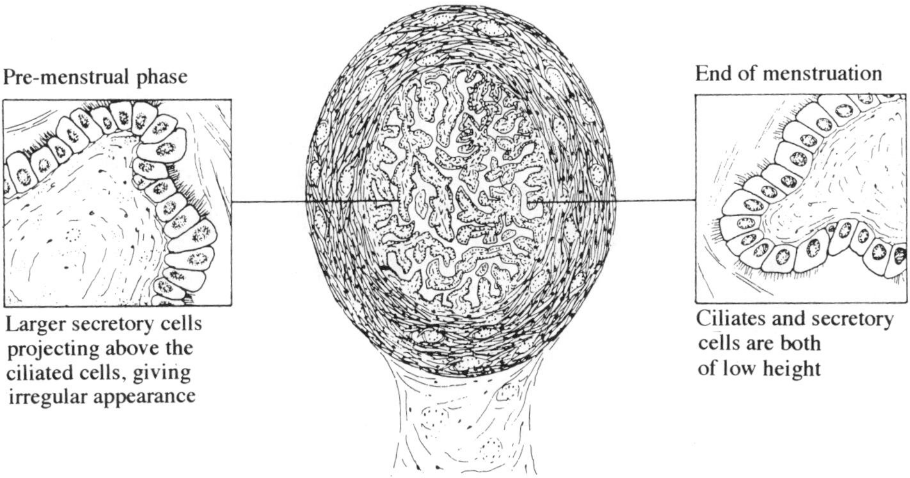

Figure 8 Changes in the Fallopian tube over the menstrual cycle

accessory sex organs and tissue. Oestrogen has a clear effect on the Fallopian tube, producing ciliated tall columnar cells and stimulating ciliary activity and secretory activity. Spontaneous muscle contractions also increase. Progesterone imposed on this oestrogen background has the opposite effect. The ciliated cells regress so that the surface becomes irregular, although the cilia are not lost (Figure 8). Secretion and muscular activity are reduced, with these changes being important for conception. The egg remains in the tube for 5 days and fertilisation takes place in the ampulla. Cell division occurs immediately, so that formation of the blastocyst occurs at the junction of the ampulla and isthmus.

The changing steroid profile produces even more marked changes in the uterus as it is first prepared to receive the transport sperm from the cervix to the Fallopian tube, and then prepares it to receive the conceptus and nourish it. As shown in Figure 9, during the oestrogen-dominated proliferation the endometrium is reconstituted. Initially the endometrium, some 2–3 mm thick, consists of stromal cells with a thin layer of small columnar cells on the luminal surface and some glandular invaginations. Under the influence of oestrogen the stroma increases, partly due to cell division and growth and partly to oedema. There is an increase both in the vascular supply to the stroma and in the number and size of the invaginations. Also increased are the height and synthetic activity of the epithelial cells, which secrete a watery fluid. At the same time myometrial activity increases.

The high oestrogen concentrations present immediately before ovulation serve to increase the number of progesterone receptors on the uterus, and the progesterone-dominated or secretory phase begins. The stroma

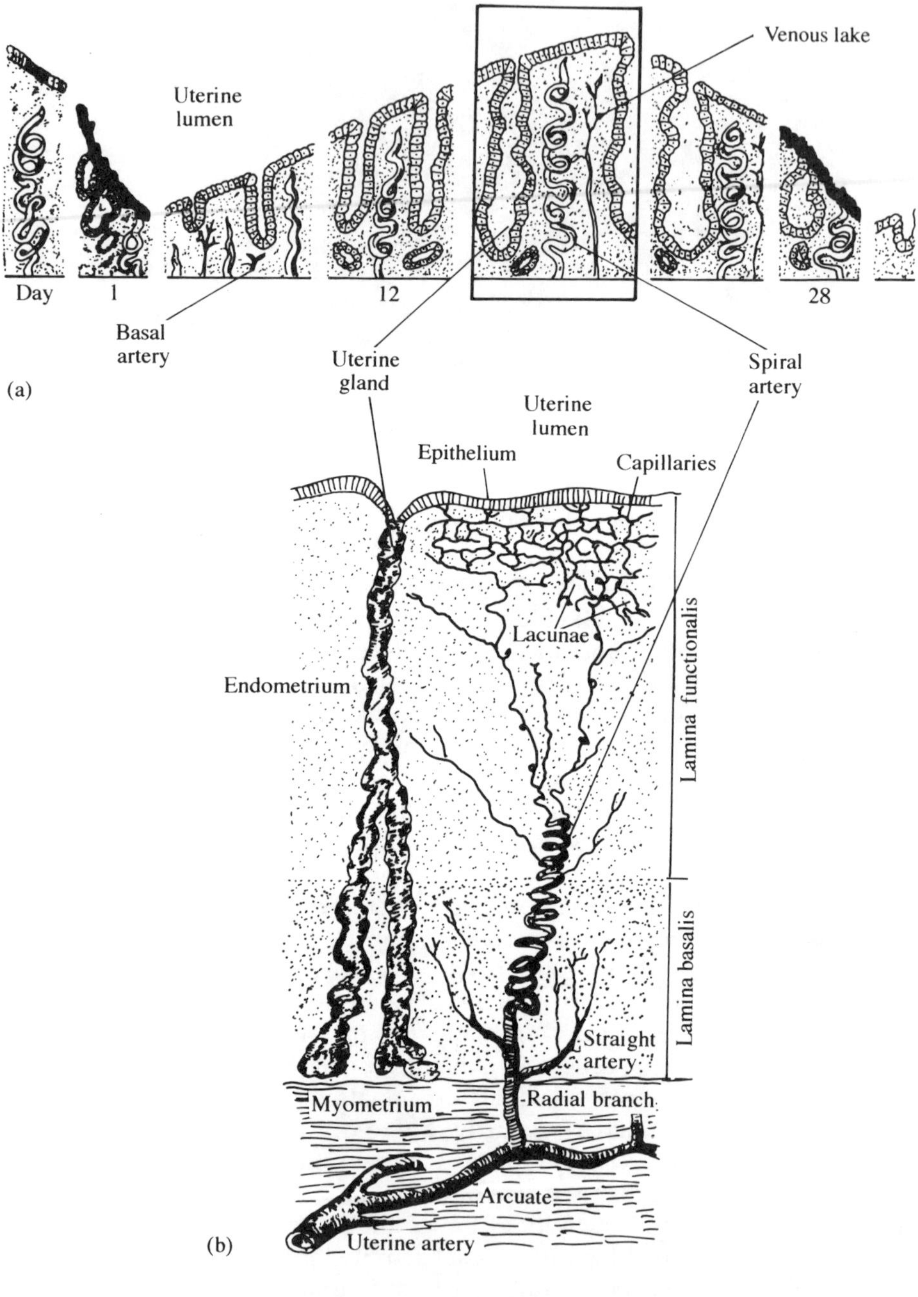

Figure 9 (a) Changes in the endometrium during the menstrual cycle. (b) Enlargement of section shown in (a)

proliferates and becomes oedematous, and the glands become convoluted and distended, with a thick secretion rich in glycoprotein. The ratio of sialomucins to sulphomucins alters during the secretory phase, which is of significance as these substances coat the epithelial cells, protecting the endometrium against infection and the action of lytic enzymes, and promoting attachment of the blastocyst. The endometrium at this stage becomes 5–6 mm thick and the blood supply to both the myometrium and endometrium increases, the vessels of the endometrium becoming coiled. Progesterone also produces enlargement of the myometrial cells and decreases excitability. There is a marked increase in enzymic activity during this phase of the cycle with, for example, an increase in lysosomal acid phosphatase, which rises as a result of an increase in the number of lysosomes in the endometrial cells.

At the end of the luteal phase, when the production of steroids falls, the secretory epithelium regresses, which adds to the coiling of the spiral arteries. There is vasoconstriction followed by vasodilation. The mechanism of the spasm of the blood vessels is not fully understood, but may involve local prostaglandins. It appears to result in necrosis of the blood vessels so that they disrupt and cause bleeding during the dilatation period. Loss of uterine debris, fluid and blood is facilitated by increased uterine contractions due to the increase in the production of prostaglandins. Menstrual blood is predominantly arterial, only 25% of the blood being of venous origin. Generally the duration of the menstrual flow is about 3–5 days, but may be as short as 1 day or as long as 8 days. The average blood loss is 30 ml, but varies from slight spotting up to 80 ml.

CHANGES IN THE VAGINA AND CERVIX

Although the cervix is continuous with the uterus, the cyclical changes are rather different. The mucosa does not undergo cyclical desquamation, but there are regular changes in the cervical mucus, which forms a barrier to infection between the vagina and uterus. Under the influence of oestrogens the cervix becomes more vascular and oedematous and produces a thinner alkaline mucus containing glycoproteins—changes which promote the survival and transport of sperm. Elongated structures forming 3 μm channels form in the mucus so that sperm can easily penetrate the cervical mucus by swimming up the channels. The beating of the flagella of the sperm produces vibration of the glycoprotein at the same frequency and this helps their progress. Cervical mucus is thinnest when oestrogen concentration is highest at mid-cycle and its elasticity or Spinnbarkeit is highest: a drop can be stretched into a thread some 8–12 cm long. At this time also, when a cervical smear is dried on a slide, a fern-like pattern develops. After ovulation, under the influence of progesterone, the mucus is greatly decreased and is thick with glycoproteins, which form a mesh-like structure that restricts penetration of the sperm. The vaginal epithelium shows characteristic changes over the monthly cycle, so that smears may be taken to determine whether it is atrophic, or under oestrogen stimulation or even to determine the presence of infections. Under the influence of oestrogen, the vaginal epithelium becomes cornified and the cells contain high concentrations of glycogen, which is broken down to lactic acid, so that the pH is low mid-cycle. Vaginal secretions also increase mid-cycle and the concentrations of metabolic substances alter, producing changes in the bacterial flora of the vagina. In monkeys these bacteria produce aliphatic acids that act as pheromones. Since the bacteria change with the cycle, these substances also change and the same could occur in the human.

CHANGES IN OTHER BODY SYSTEMS

Although full development of the mammary gland with milk production does not occur until late pregnancy and post partum, changes including some growth are seen over the menstrual cycle. The mammary gland forms a lobulated mass comprising glandular tissue, fibrous tissue connecting the lobes and adipose tissue between them (Figure 10). There are 15–20 lobes, each one being drained by a lactiferous duct that dilates into a lactiferous sinus before emerging at the nipple. The lobes themselves are subdivided into lobules, all potentially secretory and consisting of alveolar cells emptying into ducts. At birth the mammary gland consists almost entirely of lactiferous ducts and apart from a little branching the breast remains in this state until puberty, when under the influence of oestrogen the ducts develop and the ends form spherical masses of cells that subsequently develop into alveoli. After puberty oestrogens cause proliferation of mammary ducts, whereas progesterone causes growth of lobules and alveoli. Some women experience breast tenderness and swelling in the second half of the cycle, which is probably due to oedema of the interstitial tissue and distension of the ducts.

While the physiological significance of the ovarian steroids may be regarded in terms of reproduction and the effects on reproductive tissue, the steroids do affect other systems, in particular the cardiovascular system and fluid balance. Oestrogens have a significant action on plasma cholesterol, lowering it and inhibiting atherogenesis. They may thus contribute to the relatively low incidence of atherosclerotic disease and complications, such as myocardial infarction, in pre-menopausal women. In contrast, high doses of oestrogens appear to promote thrombosis by an effect on clotting factors.

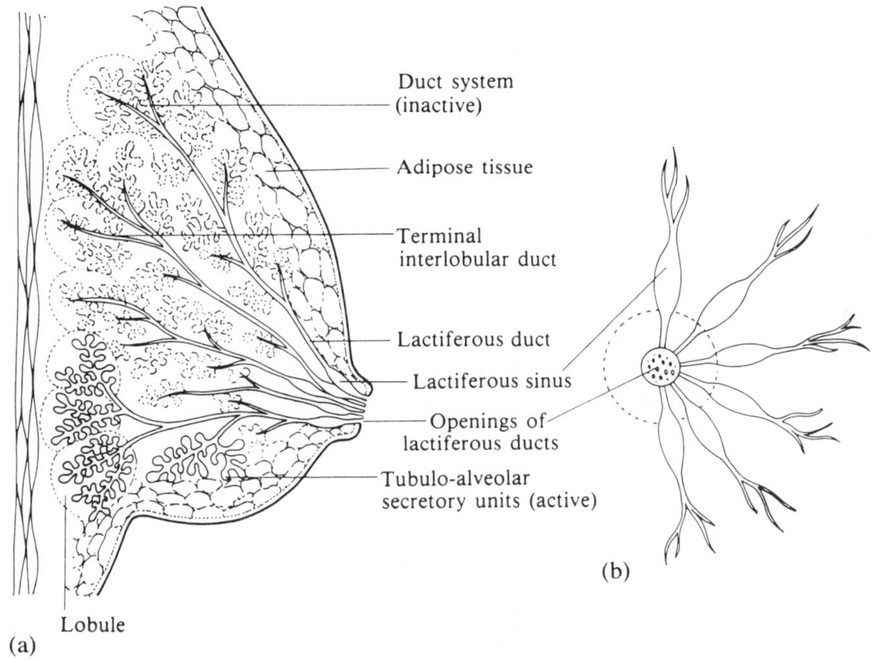

Figure 10 Structure of the mammary gland, showing (a) the general anatomy and (b) the arrangement of the duct system. Reproduced from Stanier, M.W. and Forsling, M.L. (1989). *Physiological Processes: An Introduction to Mammalian Physiology*, by permission of McGraw Hill.

They also influence haemostasis by reducing capillary fragility. The salt and water retention seen before menstruation may in part be due to the actions of oestrogen. Progesterone too can influence salt and water balance. In very large doses it produces natriuresis, probably by antagonising the action of aldosterone. Among the other actions of progesterone are a stimulatory effect on respiration and a possible thermogenic effect, body temperature increasing by 0.2–0.6°C in the days after ovulation. Concentrations of interleukin 1, which also induces fever, rise immediately after ovulation.

CONTROL OF OVARIAN FUNCTION

Ovarian function is controlled by the anterior pituitary, which in turn is controlled by the hypothalamus. Control from the hypothalamus allows for generation of a rhythm and for reproduction to be influenced by external factors. External stimuli such as day length, stress, social interaction and possibly even odours can modify secretion of anterior pituitary hormones, specifically those involved in reproduction. In man the pituitary gland comprises two lobes: the anterior or adenohypophysis and the posterior or neurohypophysis (Figure 11). In other species there is a third or intermediate lobe. The posterior lobe comprises pituicytes and nerve terminals of neurosecretory cells whose cell bodies are located in the paraventricular and supraoptic nuclei, the secretory products being oxytocin and vasopressin. The anterior pituitary comprises secretory cells arranged in irregular cords separated by vascular channels. Originally, on the basis of staining characteristics, the cells were divided into non-granular neutrophil chromophobe cells and granular chromophil cells, further subdivided into acidophils and basophils. More recently the techniques of immunofluorescence and immunocytochemistry have enabled the site of synthesis of each of the six anterior pituitary hormones to be established. Five separate functional types have been identified, LH and FSH being produced by one cell type—the gonadotrophs. They are round or polyhedral in shape and contain many dense granules approximately 200 nm in diameter.

The hormones LH and FSH, like human chorionic gonadotrophin, are glycoprotein hormones composed of two subunits: a β subunit which is hormone-specific and an α subunit which is common to these three hormones as well as TSH. The ovarian action of LH and FSH has already been described. As indicated, just before ovulation there is an increase in LH

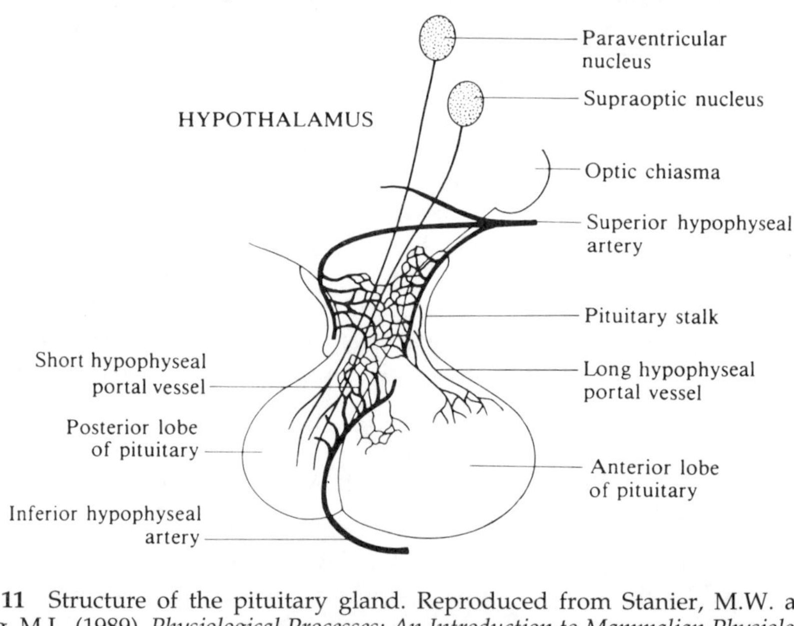

Figure 11 Structure of the pituitary gland. Reproduced from Stanier, M.W. and Forsling, M.L. (1989). *Physiological Processes: An Introduction to Mammalian Physiology*, by permission of McGraw Hill

receptors in the granulosa cells of the follicle, which in turn become steroidogenic and secrete progesterone. Post-ovulation the function of the corpus luteum is maintained by LH. FSH stimulates follicular development in the ovary and this effect is augmented by oestrogens and LH. Under the influence of the rise of FSH early in the menstrual cycle the primary follicles develop into secretory follicles. As indicated, one follicle develops to maturity, the rest undergoing atresia. It appears that the 'window' at which FSH is rising will find only one follicle at the correct stage of development.

Ovarian function thus depends on the changing pattern of pituitary gonadotrophins. Basal secretion of gonadotrophins is slightly higher during the early follicular phase than that at other times of the cycle because there is a reduced negative feedback from the ovarian steroids. The pituitary hormone levels then fall as the steroid hormones decrease, LH being more sensitive to the feedback inhibition than FSH. Inhibin output also rises as the follicle grows and this also exerts negative feedback on FSH. While oestrogens normally exert negative feedback effects both at the level of the hypothalamus and pituitary, the pre-ovulatory surge is produced by positive feedback. If concentrations increase some 200–400% more than in the early follicular phase, and remain at this high level for 48 h, then LH and FSH secretion is enhanced and then suppressed. Around 8 days after ovulation there is a peak in circulating progesterone concentrations, accompanied by a second peak in circulating oestrogens. Although oestrogen concentrations are at a relatively high level, in the presence of progesterone they have no negative feedback effect. LH, FSH, together with testosterone and inhibin, decline to their lowest level at this time.

In addition to showing characteristic changes over 28 days, LH and FSH show a series of peaks of secretion over 24 h. Thus, in the follicular phase LH is secreted in a series of low-amplitude peaks of relatively high frequency—about one per hour. On the other hand, during the luteal phase the pulses are of high amplitude and occur in an irregular fashion with intervals of up to 6 h. It appears that progesterone reduces pulse frequency, whereas oestrogen acts to reduce pulse amplitude.

Secretion of LH and FSH is thus controlled by feedback of ovarian steroids (Figure 12) and in addition by GnRH, also termed luteinising hormone-releasing hormone (LHRH), a nonapeptide synthesised in neurones lying in the hypophysiotrophic region of the hypothalamus, the axons terminating in the region of the median eminence. The releasing hormone enters into the portal circulation and is transported to the anterior pituitary, where it binds to the gonadotrophs, causing hormone release. Although there are two gonadotrophins, there appears to be only one releasing hormone and it is the most important final common mediator of all influences on reproduction conveyed through the central nervous system. GnRH is secreted in episodic bursts and it is these bursts that produce the peaks of

LH. This pulsatile secretion of GnRH is essential for the normal functioning of the gonadotrophs; a constant infusion of GnRH produces down-regulation of the anterior pituitary. The pattern of GnRH pulses can affect differential synthesis and secretion of FSH and LH. Slow-frequency pulses favour FSH synthesis. Faster pulses as seen during puberty and the late follicular phase increase LH synthesis and secretion. Thus the ability to change the pattern of GnRH stimulation of the gonadotrophin-secreting cells appears to be a mechanism which, combined with the gonadal steroids and peptides, allows a single releasing hormone to regulate differential secretion of LH and FSH. The nature and exact location of the pulse generator in the hypothalamus are unknown, although considerable information has accumulated on the neurochemical regulation of GnRH. Noradrenaline is involved, but needs only to be present occasionally to induce phasic but asynchronous activation of GnRH neurones. The neurones are then synchronised by simultaneous disinhibition of a GABAergic inhibitory tone. This seems to be the basic mechanism for uninfluenced GnRH pulsatility.

Endogenous opioid peptides, probably β-endorphins, are then able to modulate the pulsatility of GnRH neurones. Part of the steroid feedback mechanism of oestrogen and progesterone may be explained in terms of the contribution of opioid pathways. There is substantial evidence to suggest a key function for opioid peptides in the control of female reproduction. Infertility, for example, is typical in members of both sexes who abuse opiates.

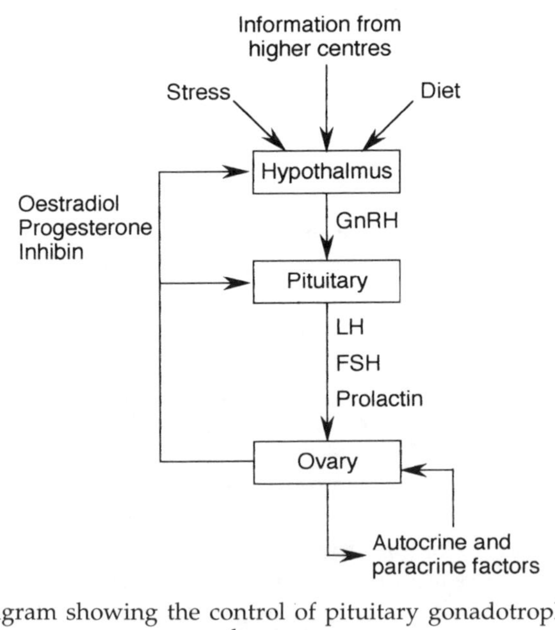

Figure 12 Diagram showing the control of pituitary gonadotrophins and ovarian hormones

Experimental studies on the effect of opioid peptides on LH release have centred on naloxone infusion. This stimulates LH secretion in a manner dependent on age. While naloxone administered to pre-pubertal children does not significantly affect LH levels, increases are seen in children at advanced stages of pubertal maturation. No response is seen in children with gonadal dysgenesis or delayed puberty or indeed in women with hypothalamic amenorrhoea. Change of opioid control of LH secretion during the menstrual cycle is also observed, the naloxone-induced rise of LH being related to circulating oestradiol levels.

These complex neuroendocrinological control mechanisms are exquisitely sensitive to general changes in both the internal and external environment as well as to changes in the endocrine environment. Loss of body weight is one such factor, be it deliberately self-induced or not. The degree to which alterations in menstruation occur on weight loss is quite variable, ranging from the amenorrhoea experienced in anorexia nervosa to oligomenorrhoea associated with, for example, bulimia or exercise programmes. Frisch's theory that a critical metabolic size or weight is required for the events of puberty to occur and regular menstruation to commence has stimulated much of the interest in weight changes and disturbances of menstruation. For the initiation of menstruation a woman must have a minimum of 17% body fat and will require 22% fat content to maintain normal menstruation. With participation by more women in strenuous exercise programmes there is an increasing awareness of the possibility of menstrual problems; up to 50% of women athletes may be affected. The underlying cause may in part be due to alterations in oestrogen metabolism induced by the loss of body weight and fat, but many other factors are involved.

In summary, understanding of the control of the menstrual cycle has increased considerably over the past few years, revealing it to be an immensely complex process. Advances have depended on the development of improved techniques particularly in the field of hormone isolation, synthesis and measurement. Much, however, still remains to be elucidated, but new tools of investigation continue to become available, including those of molecular biology.

SUGGESTED READING

Austin, C.R. and Short, R.V. (eds) (1991). *Reproduction in Mammals. Book 3: Hormonal Control of Reproduction.* Cambridge University Press, Cambridge.

Ganong, W.F. (1991). *Review of Medical Physiology.* Lange Medical Publications.

Langman, J. *Medical Embryology.* Williams & Wilkins, Baltimore.

Warwick, R. and Williams, P. *Gray's Anatomy.* Longman, London.

2

Female Puberty: Normal and Abnormal Development

Colm O'Herlihy* and D.C. Costigan†
**University College, National Maternity Hospital, Dublin, and*
†Our Lady's Hospital for Sick Children, Crumlin, Dublin, Ireland

The gradual transition of the reproductive system and its secondary physical characteristics from immaturity to a state functionally capable of reproduction is encompassed by puberty. Adolescence describes the profound contemporary psychological changes associated with this process, which have less obvious but no less important influences on the individual's functional maturity. Pubertal transition takes a number of years to complete. Its average age of onset has stabilized in the developed world since about 1960, having declined during the preceding century by an average of 4 months per decade, presumably as a result of improved childhood nutrition.

Family and twin studies suggest that pubertal age is now controlled mainly by genetic rather than nutritional influences. Dietary disturbance and adverse psychological factors can, nevertheless, all affect the timing and progress of puberty; exogenous obesity usually leads to an earlier onset. The quantity of body fat as a proportion of body mass can be significantly altered by dieting and exercise patterns in adolescents, and a critical body weight of about 47 kg has been proposed as a pre-requisite for menarche.

The normal age range for onset (9–13 years) and completion (12–17 years) is quite wide in girls, who generally complete the process 1–2 years before their male contemporaries. The acceleration in linear growth, which usually signals the start of puberty, begins and ends sooner in girls. Peak height velocity occurs in early to mid-puberty in girls, in contrast to late puberty in

---

Understanding Common Disorders in Reproductive Endocrinology. Edited by M.M. Dooley and M.P. Brincat.

boys. This results in the observed sex differences in average adult height of 12.5 cm between men and women, consequent on earlier closure of the epiphyses of female long bones.

PHYSICAL CHANGES OF PUBERTY

Thorough documentation of the physical changes of puberty by Marshall and Tanner in 1969 has led to the universal adoption of the five-stage classification of the sequence in both sexes; the female stages are summarised in Table 1. Thelarche, or breast budding, is usually the first development, coinciding with the onset of the growth spurt. The appearance of pubic hair (pubarche) occurs on average about 6 months later, and axillary hair 2 years later.

Peak growth velocity precedes the first menstruation. The average menarcheal age is 13.0 years and is followed by declining linear growth over the next 2 years. Post-menarchial cycles are often irregular and anovulatory for up to 2 years owing to immaturity of the pituitary–ovarian feedback mechanisms, and in particular the mid-cycle positive feedback relationship between oestradiol and luteinising hormone (LH) surges. This may occasionally give rise to debilitatingly heavy menstrual loss. Deposition of fat on the hips and enlargement of the bony pelvic inlet to approximate the adult female body habitus are completed before the oestrogen-induced epiphyseal closure consequent on regular menstruation.

Table 1 Stages of pubertal development in girls

Stage	Breast	Pubic hair	Age (years)
1	Pre-pubertal nipple elevation only	Nil	Prepubertal
2	Breast bud grows under areola	Sparse straight pigmented labial hair	9–13
3	Further enlargement without separation of breast and areola	Dark, coarse, curled hair sparsely over mons pubis	10–14
4	Areola and nipple elevated above breast contour	Adult-type hair abundant, but limited to mons	11–15
5	Recession of areola to contour of breast	Adult-type hair in quantity and distribution	12–17

Modified from Marshall and Tanner (1969).

ENDOCRINOLOGY OF PUBERTY

Puberty consists of two distinct hormonal processes: gonadal maturation or 'gonadarche', and adrenal androgen secretion, known as 'adrenarche'. Following a transient reactive rise in circulating gonadotrophin levels at birth due to removal of negative feedback from maternal and placental oestrogen and progesterone, follicle-stimulating hormone (FSH) and LH decline to very low circulating levels by the end of the first year and normally remain so for at least the next 8 years. This suppression during childhood is due to a central endogenous opiate suppressant mechanism which combines with an exquisitely sensitive hypothalamic–pituitary feedback centre, reactive to tiny gonadal oestrogen concentrations to maintain its 'gonadostat'. Neural inhibition of pulsatile hypothalamic gonadotrophin-releasing hormone (GnRH) secretion decreases with the approach of puberty. GnRH pulse amplitude first increases during sleep, inducing a preferential increment in LH secretion from the pituitary. Diurnal pulsatility is established by mid-puberty with an associated rise in FSH. These gonadotrophin surges invoke ovarian follicular oestradiol and inhibin responses. Positive feedback of oestrogen on the pituitary then develops and produces the mid-cycle peak of gonadotrophins typical of the adult ovulatory pattern. The external pubertal manifestations follow the hormonal maturation process. Ovarian volume increases and prolactin may also serve to enhance mammary growth. The attainment of Tanner stage 4 breast development is a widely used clinical predictor that menarche will follow within 6 months.

The adrenal cortex begins to secrete increasing amounts of dehydroepiandrosterone (DHEA) and its sulphate (DHEAS) several years before gonadarche. This secretion continues throughout puberty and is dependent on adrenocorticotrophic hormone (ACTH), with possibly another hitherto undetected pituitary hormone as an initiator. These adrenal adrogens are responsible for pubic and axillary hair development, which may precede breast growth in 15% of girls.

PRECOCIOUS PUBERTAL DEVELOPMENT

Puberty represents the normal biological transition from immature to adult reproductive functional status. The age range during which these changes take place is relatively wide, with their onset in girls normally varying between the ages of 9 and 13 years. Development is generally considered precocious when it commences before 8 years and although it is usually the result of benign constitutional early maturation, a proportion of cases are caused by a potentially serious underlying disease. Every case, therefore, needs thorough investigation and careful follow-up.

Irrespective of the cause, precocious puberty has two major deleterious consequences for the young girl. First, the period of pre-pubertal growth is considerably shortened and this, combined with an often very rapid bony maturation and premature epiphyseal fusion, results in the seeming paradox of a tall child who, without effective treatment, will become a short adult. Second, the rapid pace of hormonal change in the psychologically immature girl often results in distressing emotional outbursts, isolation from peers and occasionally the shock of unexpected menarche.

Aetiology

Precocious puberty is much commoner in girls than boys, and may commence at any age from infancy onwards. Accelerated linear growth is usually its first manifestation, followed, as in the physiological sequence, by thelarche. The growth of pubic hair (pubarche) may not occur or may be delayed. Menarche can occur at any time and parents must be warned of this possibility. An aetiological classification is described in Table 2. *Central or true precocious puberty* denotes changes consequent on normal but premature activation of the hypothalamic–pituitary–ovarian axis. In *peripheral precocious puberty (pseudo-puberty)* sexual development results from hormones arising from without the normal axis.

True central precocity can be constitutional without evidence of any disorder. This occurs close to the normal time of puberty and is often familial. Idiopathic true precocious puberty is a diagnosis of exclusion, and is much more common in girls than boys.

Several neurological disorders can induce early activation of the hypothalamic reproductive axis. Tumours such as hypothalamic hamartomas,

Table 2 Aetiological classification of precocious puberty

A	Central precocious puberty (hypothalamic–pituitary axis activated)	(i)	Constitutional/familial	5%
		(ii)	True ideopathic	70–75%
		(iii)	Central neurological lesions	5–10%
B	Precocious pseudo-puberty (normal endocrine axis inactive)	(i)	McCune–Albright syndrome	5%
		(ii)	Functioning ovarian cysts and tumours	5%
		(iii)	Adrenal hyperplasia/tumours	Rare
		(iv)	Gonadotrophins from gonadal tumours	Rare
		(v)	Chronic hypothyroidism	Rare
		(vi)	Exogenous sex steroid ingestion	

astrocytomas, ependymomas and gliomas; previous central nervous system (CNS) insults such as hydrocephalus, cranial irradiation, CNS infections or skull trauma may all induce precocious development (Figure 1). All cause early release from central inhibition of the endocrine axis and must be considered in the differential diagnosis. Chronic hypothyroidism is thought to induce central precocious puberty by thyroid-stimulating hormone (TSH)/LH overlap.

Peripheral precocious pseudo-puberty is most often caused by oestrogen emanating from a source other than physiologically activated follicular function. McCune–Albright syndrome refers to polyostotic fibrous dysplasia,

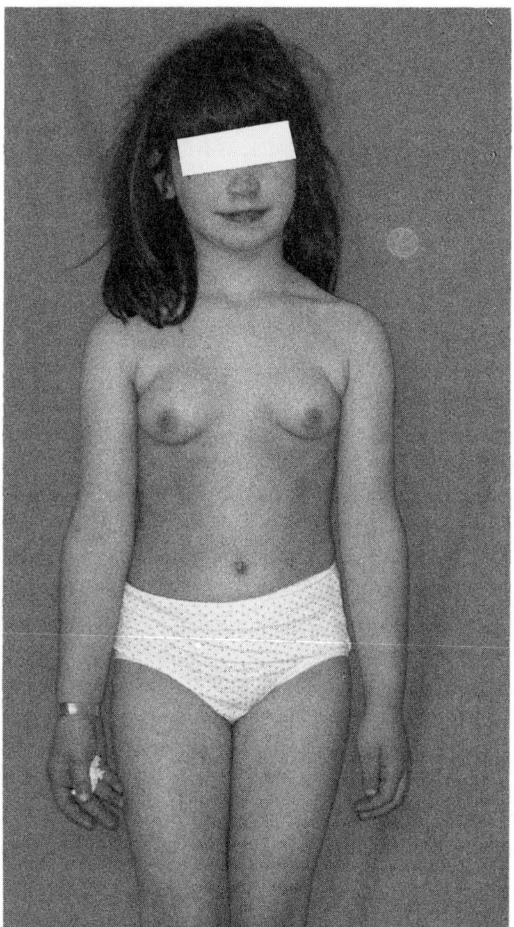

Figure 1 Central precocious puberty secondary to a hypothalamic hamartoma. Chronological age = 6 years; bone age = 9.5 years

characterised by multiple cystic lesions of the skull and long bones, a propensity to fracture, café-au-lait skin patches, and a predisposition to other endocrine hypersecretion disorders. In most girls the precocious puberty is peripheral due to autonomous follicular function. Some follicular cysts secrete enough oestrogen to induce precocious puberty. Theca granulosa tumours of the ovary and gonadoblastomas may do likewise and cause vaginal bleeding to occur disproportionately early in the developmental sequence in association with an abdominopelvic mass. Some adrenal tumours are said to feminise rather than virilise but are very rare. Exogenous oestrogen either through ingestion of medications, such as contraceptive pills, or eating meat from oestrogen-treated animals should not be forgotten as an occasional source of exposure.

Evaluation of precocious puberty

A good clinical history is required to elucidate the duration and speed of progression of the precocity, the presence of a predisposing personal or family history and the impact of the condition upon the girl. A careful physical examination should document the Tanner stage of puberty, and to check for neurological or pelvic lesions. Ultrasound examination can confirm ovarian and uterine enlargement and detect ovarian or adrenal cysts or masses. A standard X-ray of left wrist and hand for bone age is crucial to confirm the precocious bone maturation and to evaluate the pace of progression; this can be repeated serially every 3–6 months, to monitor the effects of therapy (Table 3).

Hormonal evaluation is needed to differentiate central from peripheral causes of precocious puberty. Because FSH and LH release is pulsatile,

Table 3 Investigation of precocious puberty

1 Serial documentation of growth and development, using Tanner charts

2 Neurological and abdominopelvic examination

3 Radiology:
- (i) pelvic ultrasound
- (ii) serial left hand/wrist for bone age
- (iii) skull and pituitary fossa X-ray
  or
- (iv) computed tomography or magnetic resonance imaging of head

4 Endocrinology:
- (i) Basal FSH, LH, oestradiol, human chorionic gonadotrophin
- (ii) GnRH stimulation test
- (iii) Thyroid function tests
- (iv) DHEAS, testosterone if virilisation

circulating oestrogen levels may be very low and basal values are often not discriminatory. In central precocity, however, LH release in response to GnRH stimulation (the GnRH test) is in the pubertal range or greater, whereas peripheral causes are not associated with enhanced LH output because the unstimulated pituitary gonadotrophin cells have synthesised very little pre-formed LH. Girls with the elevated or pubertal response pattern to GnRH require either computed tomography of the hypothalamic area to include coronal views or magnetic resonance imaging to exclude a developing neurological lesion.

Management of precocious puberty

The vast majority of girls with precocious puberty have a central idiopathic variety and thus treatment must be symptomatic. The urgency of treatment depends on the pace of progression of the pubertal process, bearing in mind that spontaneous cessation of precocity may sometimes occur. Fortunately, in recent years both precocious sexual and osseous development can be halted using analogues of GnRH with superagonist activity that 'down-regulate' the pituitary responsiveness to endogenous pulsatile GnRH and effect a reversible interruption of hypothalamic stimulation of the pituitary–gonadal axis; this inhibition is reversible. Stable levels of GnRH agonists are preferable and best achieved using slow-release depot, subcutaneous or intramuscular preparations given at monthly intervals. Their effectiveness can be assessed by serial GnRH testing and, more usually, by documenting clinical regression in Tanner staging and slowing of the rate of bone maturity. Ideally, therapy is continued until either bone age matches chronological age or until 12 years and cessation is followed by prompt restarting of the normal pubertal transition. Subsequent fertility and age of menopause are not altered in women who have undergone central precocious puberty.

Peripheral (pseudo)-precocious puberty due to inappropriate oestrogen secretion is difficult to correct effectively. Ovarian masses, such as theca–granulosa tumours, should be treated by oophorectomy; conservative attempts at enucleation of the abnormal tissue may later be followed by recurrence. Follicular cysts can be confidently identified by ultrasound and aspirated either percutaneously or via laparoscopy; this is usually curative once the causative stimulus has been removed.

Incomplete precocity can occasionally occur with early thelarche, pubarche or menarche alone and without progression to the other pubertal changes. Premature thelarche most often occurs in girls under 3 years who may have been born pre-term, and is not associated with progression to the other pubertal changes.

Isolated pubarche/adrenarche, with development of pubic hair and axillary odour, is normal after 6 years of age in girls. No oestrogen effect is obvious in breast or vaginal mucosa but there may be slight acceleration of growth and bony maturation. Pubarche/adrenarche in younger girls or with more than minimal androgen effects should suggest investigation for excess androgen secretion, such as in late-onset congenital adrenal hyperplasia. Isolated premature menarche may present without other signs of sexual development and may cease spontaneously, but all other causes of precocious oestrogen secretion need to be excluded.

DELAYED PUBERTY

Delayed puberty by definition occurs when its onset is delayed more than 2.5 SD from the mean of 13 years. Moreover, the progress of some girls through the pubertal changes is abnormally slow and this may also warrant investigation, as when no menarche has occurred within 5 years of onset of puberty. The causes of delayed female puberty are outlined in Table 4. In practice, the absence of any developmental signs and especially of thelarche by the age of 14 years will include fewer than 5% of the normal adolescent population; many parents, nevertheless, seek advice about their daughters' infantile features before this age. The problem is an uncommon one in the absence of chronic debilitative illness and its most common cause, gonadal failure, is not correctable.

Constitutional delay is most often associated with a delay in growth and bone maturation. The pubertal stage correlates with bone age, and height,

Table 4 Commoner causes of delayed puberty

Cause		Serum gonadotrophins
Constitutional/idiopathic	15%	Low/normal
Gonodal failure Turner's syndrome Pure gonadal dysgenesis Non-dysgenetic failure	45%	Elevated
Hypothalamic–pituitary dysfunction CNS tumours, infections, malformations Deficient gonadotrophins, e.g. Kallmann's syndrome, pituitary insufficiency	25%	Low
Defective steroid synthesis	5%	Low
Other disorders (including chronic illness, malnutrition)	10%	Low

although short, is usually appropriate for the family when expressed as a function of bone age. Growth rate is normal for bone age and puberty commences usually at a bone age of 11 years. This pattern of development is often familial, with mother or older sisters also experiencing delayed menarche. Girls who have had significant intercurrent illness during childhood which has delayed skeletal growth and osseous maturation may also begin puberty later. The prognosis for later reproductive function is normal in these cases.

Hypergonatrophic hypogonadism implies a normal hypothalamo–pituitary attempt to stimulate abnormal ovaries. Turner's syndrome, a sporadic disorder occurring in one in 2500 female births, is the commonest example of this form of delayed puberty. It is always associated with short stature, which is growth hormone responsive and should be diagnosed before delayed puberty becomes a problem. The cause is a complete or partial absence of one of the X chromosomes.

Approximately 50% have 45X0 genotype. Mosaicism (usually 45X0/46XX) is present in 30–40%. Because the classical clinical features of short neck, low hairline, high palate, hypoplastic wide-spaced nipples, broad chest, cubitus valgus and lymphoedema are most strongly associated with the 45X0 genotype, many girls with Turner's syndrome only exhibit short stature and gonadal dysgenesis ('streak ovaries'). A karyotype, therefore, should be performed on all girls in this category. Some girls with a mosaic XX line may have enough ovarian function to respond to the very high gonadotrophin levels by producing enough oestrogen to initiate pubertal development, but this function fails in later puberty or in the early twenties, leading to a premature menopausal picture. Primary ovarian failure may also occur in girls whose ovaries are damaged by radiation or chemotherapy for malignant disease or by autoantibodies in syndromes such as Addison's disease.

Pure gonadal dysgenesis is associated with a normal genotype, streak ovaries and a female phenotype, which includes normal Müllerian-derived internal female organs. An XY form may be incomplete, so that some testosterone may emanate from the streak gonads. All forms of XY gonadal dysgenesis need bilateral gonadectomy (even prior to puberty) to prevent the development of gonadoblastoma in 5–20% in later years.

Hypogonadotrophic hypogonadism due to isolated gonadotrophin deficiency may be a sporadic or autosomally inherited condition. The coexistence of anosmia or hyposmia constitutes Kallmann's syndrome. These girls are of normal height but may have a decreased upper/lower segment ratio. It can be very difficult to differentiate isolated gonadotrophin deficiency from constitutional delay in puberty without a prolonged period of observation, which may be psychologically unacceptable to the adolescent girl.

The coexistence of other hypothalamic–pituitary hormone deficiency, such as growth hormone deficiency, points to the aetiology of hypogonadotrophic hypogonadism. This may be associated with midline abnormalities such as cleft lip/palate or optic nerve hypoplasia in some cases. Tumours in the region of the pituitary fossa, such as craniopharyngioma or glioma or their treatment with surgery or radiation, may also damage the pituitary source of LH and FSH. Miscellaneous hypothalamic abnormalities such as Laurence–Moon–Biedl syndrome or the reversible hypothalamic disturbance seen in anorexia nervosa, severe intercurrent illness or malnutrition with weight loss to less than 80% of ideal body weight may also lead to hypogonadotrophic dysfunction.

Differential diagnosis

Diagnostic evaluation is helped by historical clues such as lymphoedema at birth, significant childhood illness, evidence of other hormone deficiency or an abnormal sense of smell. The family history should be assessed for the timing of puberty, parental heights and infertility in relatives. Clinical examination should include height and weight, breast palpation (to check if Tanner stage 2 breast budding is present), a search for stigmata of Turner's syndrome, an evaluation of smell function and a careful neurological examination, including fundoscopy and visual field perimetry. X-ray of the left wrist and hand can be very helpful because, if puberty is significantly delayed for bone age, then constitutional delay is unlikely. Measurement of serum LH and FSH is mandatory, as is a karyotype in all girls with elevated values. A pubertal GnRH test may predict the onset of pubertal development by a year or more and may be very useful to differentiate constitutional delay from those with hypogonadotrophic hypogonadism.

Treatment

Treatment is not normally indicated for constitutional delay of puberty other than explanation and reassurance for the patient and her parents. Occasionally, if the girl is suffering psychologically or if there is considerable delay or inability to confirm this diagnosis, a 3-month trial of oestrogen therapy, such as ethinyloestradiol, may produce enough breast development to reassure the child, and usually this is soon followed by spontaneous puberty.

Theoretically, in girls with hypogonadotrophism, pubertal development and ovulatory menstruation can be induced using pulsatile GnRH via a subcutaneous infusion pump or with exogenous gonadotrophin injections. However, because of the technical difficulties and expense of such treatment, secondary sexual development is usually induced with exogenous oestrogens, followed by later introduction of progestagens in both the hypo- and hypergonadotrophic varieties of pubertal delay. A suggested regimen begins with ethinyloestradiol 2–4 μg per day (or Premarin 0.625 mg per day), followed by a gradually increasing dose during the subsequent 2 years, while regularly monitoring the effect on growth velocity, breast and areolar development and bone maturation. Excessively rapid increments in dosage can result in disproportionate (and unsightly) areolar development or permanent loss of height potential through excessive bone stimulation. Once an ethinyloestradiol dosage of over 10 μg per day is reached, breakthrough bleeding is likely to occur unless a progestagen is introduced in a cyclic fashion for about 10–12 days per month.

The normality of external and internal genitalia must be emphasised to girls with delayed puberty. Moreover, those with permanent hypogonadotrophic hypogonadism (and their parents) need reassurance about their later ability to ovulate following stimulation with pulsatile GnRH or exogenous gonadotrophins. Girls with hypergonadotrophic hypogonadism can be informed of the possibility of future successful pregnancy resulting from oocyte donation and fertilisation followed by intrauterine embryo transfer and endometrial implantation.

Throughout what is usually a long investigative and treatment process, all these patients and their relatives require continuing psychological support and explanation appropriate to their chronological age. Once a rapport has been established, a regular review of progress is worth while on at least a yearly basis extending into adulthood, so as to provide an opportunity for counselling on subsequent reproductive options.

SUGGESTED READING

Dewhurst, J. (1984). *Female Puberty and its Abnormalities.* Churchill Livingstone, Edinburgh.

Manasco, P. K., Pescovitz, O. H., Hill, S. C. *et al.* (1989). Six-year results of lutenizing hormone releasing hormone (LHRH) agonist treatment in children with LHRH-dependent precocious puberty. *J. Pediatr.*, **115**, 105–108.

Marshall, W. A. and Tanner, J. M. (1969). Variations in the pattern of pubertal changes in girls. *Arch. Dis. Child.*, **44**, 291–303.

Speroff, L., Glass, R. H. and Kase, N. G. (eds) (1992). *Clinical Gynaecologic Endocrinology and Infertility*, 4th edn. Williams and Wilkins, Baltimore; see especially Ch. 13: Abnormal puberty and growth problems, pp. 363–292.

Wheeler, M. D. and Styne, D. M. (1990). Diagnosis and management of precocious puberty. *Pediatr. Clin. North Am.*, **37**, 1255–1271.

3

Menstrual Disorders and Endometriosis

Michael M. Dooley
West Dorset Hospital, Dorchester, UK

DYSFUNCTIONAL UTERINE BLEEDING

Menstrual blood loss has a skewed distribution with a mean of 35 ml and a 90th centile of 80 ml. Menstrual blood loss in excess of 80 ml is considered pathological. Without treatment such a loss will lead to iron-deficiency anaemia and constitute objective menorrhagia.

Definitions

Dysfunctional uterine bleeding is defined as excessive or prolonged regular menstrual bleeding in the absence of overt uterine, endocrine or haematological disorder.

Menorrhagia is defined as excessive menstrual bleeding that occurs with irregular or regular cycles.

Incidence

In 1985, 18 600 hysterectomies were performed for menstrual disorders in England. Thirty per 1000 consultations with general practitioners are for excessive menstrual bleeding.

Pathophysiology

Abnormal menstrual bleeding may be ovulatory or anovulatory. As a rule of thumb irregular prolonged cycles are associated with anovulation, and

Understanding Common Disorders in Reproductive Endocrinology. Edited by M.M. Dooley and M.P. Brincat.

regular cycles are associated with ovulation. Anovulation is more common around puberty and the climacteric. About 20% of women who present with menstrual dysfunction will have anovulatory cycles.

The cause of bleeding in anovulatory cycles is usually due to the imbalance of oestrogen and progesterone, with the stimulation of the endometrium being by unopposed oestrogen. This leads to abnormal endometrial development and irregular heavy bleeding.

Ovulatory abnormal menstrual loss is more prevalent in parous women between the ages of 30 and 45 years and is characterised by heavy but regular loss. Hormonal cyclicity is thus normal. Prostaglandins (PGs) of the two series are synthesised by the endometrium and are thought to play a role in the pathology. PGE_2, PGI_2 and PGD_2 are involved with vasodilation of blood vessels and antiplatelet aggregation, while $PGF_{2\alpha}$ causes platelet aggregation and vasoconstriction. As these are mediators in the regulation of blood loss an imbalance may cause dysfunctional bleeding.

Heavy menstrual loss can also develop with an increase in the surface area of the cavity, with heavy losses occurring the greater the surface area.

Aetiology

Physiological

Pathological menstrual loss is by definition stated to occur with losses greater than 80 ml. Interpretation by the patient of her loss may be excessive and this often occurs when she has high expectations. This situation occurs more frequently around puberty and when the woman discontinues the oral contraceptive pill.

Increase in endometrial surface area

- Neoplastic, e.g. fibroids.
- Congenital, e.g. bicornuate uterus.

Infective

- Examples: endometritis; chronic pelvic inflammatory disease.

Haematological

Blood dyscrasias such as thrombocytopenia and von Willebrand's disease are associated with increased menstrual blood loss, thus suggesting that platelet dysfunction may cause menorrhagia. Long-term anticoagulant use may also cause a problem.

Metabolic

- Example: thyroid disorders.

Psychological factors

The finely tuned hypothalamic–pituitary–gonadal axis can easily be disturbed, which may lead to anovulation, e.g. the stress associated with examinations.

Traumatic

- Example: intrauterine contraceptive device.

Dysfunctional uterine bleeding is diagnosed by exclusion of the above causes.

Diagnosis

History and examination with appropriate investigations remain the cornerstone of diagnosis.

History

The changing status of women within society has led to an altered acceptance of menstrual symptoms. Younger women are less tolerant of increasing menstrual loss than older women. Although a woman's complaint may be genuine, her perception of an increased loss can be modified by other factors, including emotional upset, marital problems or even fear of genital cancer. Important historical points include:

- Sudden change in menstrual loss.
- Development of large, well-defined clot.
- Pain with the passage of clot (clot colic).
- Duration of loss is important to assess but there is no true correlation between duration of menstruation and total menstrual loss.
- Flooding.
- Frequent soiling.
- Social mishaps.
- Tiredness and lethargy (associated with anaemia).

History may be unreliable but most women would not generally wish for gynaecological examination without reason and thus it is commonly assumed to be a genuine complaint.

Examination

A general examination is important, especially looking for signs of anaemia and other endocrine disturbance. Weight is important, with adipose tissue being known to upset the oestrogen balance. A full pelvic examination to exclude fibroids or possibly an ovarian tumour and a speculum examination to exclude local causes of vaginal bleeding, e.g. cervical carcinoma, is essential.

Investigations

These include:

- Full blood count.
- Thyroid function test.
- Clotting profile if clotting disorders are suspected from the history.
- Endocervical swab if infection is suspected from the history.
- Is she ovulating or not? A clinical diagnosis of anovulatory dysfunctional uterine bleeding may be made with reasonable accuracy on history alone, taking into account the patient's age and cycle regularity. For research purposes this needs to be confirmed by endometrial biopsy (to demonstrate secretory changes) or mid-luteal phase progesterone measurements.
- Menstrual calendar prospective approach: several methods have been developed. These include a subjective menstrual calendar recording the numbers of pads used as well as the patient's assessment.

  Another method of assessment is a pictorial blood loss assessment chart (PBAC) (see Figure 1), which can be used to assess menstrual blood loss. A close correlation has been demonstrated between menstrual blood loss and PBAC score. When menorrhagia is complained of in the presence of completely normal blood loss this chart may assist in reassurance and thus avoid unnecessary intervention.
- Objective blood loss measurement: this is needed in certain cases to help reassure the individual and thus avoid unnecessary intervention, as well as for research studies. Parental pressure may also play a role in the need for this level of assessment.

  Methods include:
  1. Weight of tampons pre- and post-use.
  2. Radioisotopic assessment of peripheral circulation pre- and post-menstruation.
  3. Iron determination: the iron content of the sanitary towel and tampons is proportional to the blood retained within them and can be determined by a variety of techniques.
  4. Haemoglobin content of menstrual blood loss.

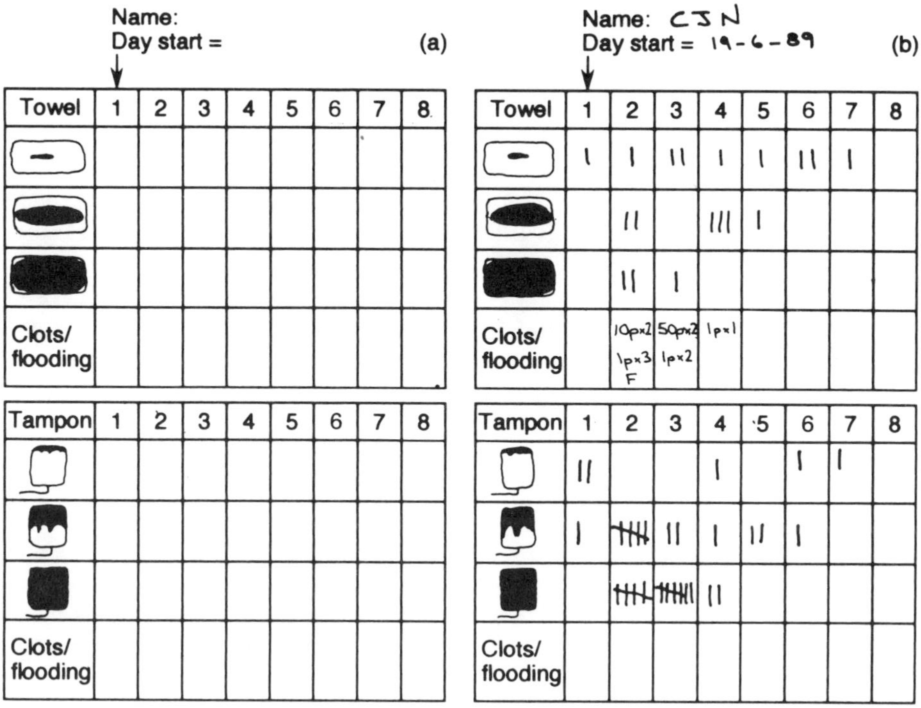

Figure 1 (a) PBAC and (b) PBAC filled in by a menorrhagic patient. From Shaw, 1990b, by permission of Parthenon Press

- Ultrasound scanning can be useful to confirm the diagnosis of fibroids and exclude gross ovarian pathology. Ultrasonic assessment of uterine volume or endometrial thickness demonstrates no significant correlation with menstrual blood loss.
- Endometrial biopsy and hysteroscopy: the immediate investigation of a dilatation and curettage should be resisted. Consideration needs to take place about what is the possible pathology and how is it best to diagnose this. Hysteroscopy allows careful assessment of the cavity and properly directed biopsy to occur.

  As a general rule an endometrial biopsy, ideally in conjunction with hysteroscopy, should be performed if heavy periods are a sudden and a recent problem (not associated with discontinuation of the oral contraceptive), if the woman is over 35 years of age or if inter-menstrual bleeding coexists.

  Formal dilatation and curettage requires a general anaesthetic but outpatient techniques can now be employed. Such methods include Vabra curettage and Gynocheck with or without outpatient hysteroscopy.

- Plasma hormone levels: gonadotrophin levels may be useful if the patient has menopausal symptoms and she may be entering the climacteric. There is a limited role in assessment of oestradiol or progesterone levels.

Treatment

Explanation and a discussion as to the patient's understanding of the problem and different treatments available are an essential part of any treatment programme. There are many misconceptions and fixed views held by patients and time spent at the beginning can be invaluable. After careful assessment any pathology found, e.g. hypothyroidism, should be appropriately treated. If the patient has an intrauterine contraceptive device *in situ* removal of this requires careful assessment of future contraceptive needs.

The treatment of fibroids again depends on the extent of the problem, including the size of the lesions and the future contraceptive needs. Fibroids can be shrunk in size temporarily with luteinising hormone-releasing hormone, which induces a reversible menopause. This reduction in size can be useful pre-operatively but as a long-term treatment is of limited effect as well as having long-term osteoporotic complications.

Once appropriate pathology has been diagnosed and dealt with the main area for treatment is dysfunctional uterine bleeding.

Medical treatment of dysfunctional uterine bleeding

This will be discussed under the two headings of anovulatory and ovulatory dysfunctional bleeding. It needs to be borne in mind that few patients at the extremes of reproductive age are consistently anovulatory or ovulatory; also all anovulatory cycles are not menorrhagic—often quite the reverse. All medical treatments for this condition are not curative and are only therefore treating the symptoms.

- Anovulatory dysfunctional uterine bleeding.
  1. *Oral contraceptive pill.* The periods will usually become lighter, more regular and less painful with the use of the oral contraceptive pill.
  2. *Progestagens.* These inhibit endometrial proliferation and induce secretory transformation. Progestagen exposure from early in the menstrual cycle will cause a thinner endometrium than normal, resulting in less blood loss. Continued long-term exposure of the endometrium to progestagens results in inhibition or suppression of secretory change and the end result is very similar histologically to atrophy. Four regimes of progestagens can be given in the treatment of dysfunctional uterine bleeding:
     (a) Days 16–25, luteal replacement: e.g. medroxyprogesterone acetate 10 mg twice a day, norithesterone 5 mg twice a day or dydrogesterone 10 mg twice a day.

(b) Days 5–25, endometrial growth reduction: this regime may also be beneficial with ovulatory dysfunctional bleeding.
(c) Continuous endometrial suppression: high-dose continual treatment has side-effects, including weight gain, nausea, bloating ankle oedema, headaches, depression, loss of libido, acne, hirsutism and upset in carbohydrate and lipid metabolism.

Therapy should be reviewed initially after 3–4 months of treatment for results of therapy, side-effects and blood pressure. After 12 months of treatment the situation needs to be fully reviewed before continuation of long-term therapy.

A progestagen causes a withdrawal bleed on an oestrogen-primed endometrium and if the woman does not experience a withdrawal bleed then there is no oestrogen stimulation of the endometrium and combination hormone replacement therapy may need to be considered.

3. *Hormone replacement therapy.* If the woman is experiencing menopausal symptoms with heavy periods then a trial of combination hormone replacement therapy needs to be considered.

- Ovulatory dysfunctional uterine bleeding.
  1. *Prostaglandin synthetase inhibitors (PGSIs).* These are non-steroidal anti-inflammatory analgesics, and a full list can be seen in Table 1.

  PGSIs, including mefenamic acid, diclofenac sodium, ibuprofen and naproxen have been shown to be effective in reducing excessive menstrual bleeding in women with intrauterine devices. Dysfunctional bleeding studies have been confined to mefenamic acid. Mefenamic acid, 500 mg three times daily during menstruation, effectively reduces menstrual blood loss in approximately 50% of patients with subjectively assessed excessive bleeding, and in 33% of cases with objectively established menorrhagia.

  Overall patient acceptability is enhanced by the drug's beneficial effect on dysmenorrhoea and other menstrually related symptoms. Mefenamic acid is only needed for 2–5 days of each cycle and thus avoids any potentially serious complications from long-term use.

Table 1 Non-steroidal anti-inflammatory analgesics

1. Aryl carboxylic acids
   (a) Salicylic acids, e.g. aspirin
   (b) Fenamates, e.g. flufenamic acid, mefenamic acid, sodium meclofenamate
2. Aryl alkanoic acids
   (a) Aryl propionic acids, e.g. ibuprofen, ketoprofen, naproxen
   (b) Indole acetic acids, e.g. indomethacin
   (c) Penylacetic acids, e.g. diclofenac sodium

Their precise mode of action is unclear but they inhibit the synthesis of cyclical endoperoxides in the microsomal fraction of the cell through their inhibitory action on the enzyme cytooxygenase.

2. *Oral contraceptive pill.* As indicated above this can be a very effective treatment as long as there are no contraindications. Endometrial growth is reduced, as is menstrual loss.
3. *Progestagens.* The endometrial growth suppression level may have a role in certain cases. Little quantitative data exist to support this treatment regime, although it is often the first line of treatment.
4. *Danazol.* This is an isoxazol derivative of 17α-ethinyltestosterone. The actions of danazol, which is dose-related, include:
   (a) Alteration of pulsatile gonadotrophin release.
   (b) Inhibition of the mid-cycle gonadotrophin surge. This leads to:
   (c) Inhibition of normal follicular maturation and growth.
   (d) Suppression of 17β-oestradiol production.
   (e) Atrophic changes in the endometrium.

   Danazol at 200 mg (some patients need 400 mg) daily will significantly reduce menstrual blood loss when administered for at least 3 months. Dysmenorrhoea is also improved with these doses.

   Side-effects with danazol appear to be dose-related, i.e. a much greater incidence is noted in the higher doses (800 mg daily) sometimes used to treat endometriosis. These side-effects include weight gain, tiredness, skeletal pain, headaches, acne and irritability. To reduce these side-effects it is important to keep the dose of danazol down to a minimum.

   Danazol does not affect the coagulation system, which makes it a safe alternative to other synthetic steroids in women over the age of 40 years.
5. *Antifibrinolytic therapy.* Antifibrinolytics act by reducing the enhanced fibrinolytic activity found in the uterus of women with excessive menstrual blood loss. They have the advantage that they need only to be taken during actual loss. Reduction of blood loss of up to 50% has been reported. Side-effects are common and these include nausea and dizzy spells.
6. *Luteinising hormone-releasing hormone analogues (GnRHa).* GnRHa are well-tolerated drugs that control dysfunctional uterine bleeding and to a lesser extent excessive menses associated with fibroids. Their effects are short lived and only really working while therapy continues. Prolonged treatment is prohibited because of the long-term side-effects, especially osteoporosis.

   GnRHa have a short-term role in the treatment of menorrhagia, perhaps while the patient awaits surgery, or a spontaneous menopause.

Surgical treatment

- *Endometrial ablation.* The aim of this treatment is to destroy the endometrium and produce a therapeutic type of Asherman's syndrome. This technique, now beginning to gain a high level of acceptance, includes laser ablation and endometrial diathermy or resection. These are carried out under direct vision. These techniques are only suitable for women who have completed their family, in whom the endometrium is histologically normal and the uterine cavity is not grossly enlarged.

  Ablation is an attractive alternative to both long-term drug treatment and hysterectomy for the management of abnormal menstruation. It is of particular use for those women who have regular, painless, heavy periods. With the use of the hysteroscope the hospital stay is shorter, recovery faster and there are thus obvious financial savings.
- *Hysterectomy.* This is the definitive treatment but does involve the risk of major surgery. The route may be vaginal or abdominal. The abdominal approach allows the ovaries to be removed with ease.

  Removal of the ovaries needs to be fully discussed pre-operatively. The following points need to be discussed with the patient:

  1. The risk of ovarian carcinoma occurring if the ovaries are left *in situ*.
  2. The risk of benign ovarian growths occurring.
  3. If the ovaries are left *in situ* pre-menstrual syndrome will still occur if it is already present or may develop in future.
  4. The menopause occurs earlier after hysterectomy owing to earlier ovarian failure.
  5. Hormone replacement therapy will be needed if the ovaries are removed (unless already menopausal).
  6. Certain women get residual ovarian pain if the ovaries are conserved.

  The use of the laparoscope and the application of autosutures is now being investigated and may allow more to be performed by the vaginal route. The vaginal route has less operative morbidity when compared to the abdominal route.

  A comparison of hysterectomy and hysteroscopic endometrial destruction is shown in Table 2.

Summary

This common complaint is due to a partially understood pathophysiology. The cornerstone of management is a thorough history with examination and limited investigation. Medical treatment, if acceptable, has a role although a lot of treatment regimes have not been fully evaluated. Minimal invasive surgery is beginning to play a much larger role in the treatment programme.

Table 2 Comparison between hysterectomy and hysteroscopic endometrial destruction

	Total hysterectomy	Endometrial surgery
Menstruation	Amenorrhoea certain	50% will menstruate
Type of surgery	Major	Minor
Hospital stay	5–7 days	1–3 days
Scars	Yes (unless vaginal)	No
Removal of ovaries	Yes	No
Rest of abdominal contents can be inspected	Yes	No
Convalescence	6–8 weeks	2–3 weeks
Risk of uterine/cervical cancer	Nil	Yes

Hysterectomy should really be considered once all other treatment options have been evaluated and fully discussed with the patient.

ENDOMETRIOSIS

Endometriosis is a commonly encountered condition of the reproductive aged female. Use of the laparoscope has demonstrated that endometriosis has various manifestations and may even be present in an otherwise normal peritoneum. It has been argued that ectopic endometrium may be physiological and only considered to be pathological if associated with symptoms or signs of progression and tissue damage.

Many aspects of the pathophysiology and treatment still remain controversial.

Definition

Endometriosis is the presence of functional endometrial tissue outside the uterine cavity. In order to confirm this histologically there must be confirmation of the presence of glands and stroma.

Adenomyosis occurs when endometrial tissue lies within the myometrium and is thus a histological diagnosis made after hysterectomy (usually for heavy periods). It is very unusual for endometriosis and adenomyosis to occur together, implying a different pathophysiology.

Incidence

There is an increasing incidence with age, with a peak between the ages of 40 and 44. This probably works out that about 10% of menstruating Caucasians have endometriosis. They may be totally asymptomatic and be an incidental finding (e.g. at laparoscopic sterilisation) or may have marked symptoms. The extent of the disease is not correlated to the symptoms.

With a significant number of women having asymptomatic endometriosis it has therefore been proposed that it may even be a clinically normal finding in certain individuals.

Pathogenesis

Several theories have been developed, including metaplasia of the coelomic epithelium. Much greater support and evidence is accumulating for the transplantation hypothesis, although no single theory answers all the questions raised.

The transplantation hypothesis proposes that endometriosis originates from uterine endometrial tissue and is transported to ectopic locations, where it implants and grows. This transportation is usually via retrograde menstruation, although vascular and lymphatic spread may play a role.

Evidence in favour of the transplantation hypothesis includes:

1. Total duration of oral contraceptive use is significantly greater in women with a normal pelvis compared to those with endometriosis.
2. Higher rates of disease with increasing intervals since last pregnancy in parous women.
3. Development of endometriosis in infertile women previously found to have no disease by laparoscopy.
4. Risk of disease less with increased number of births, later menarche and irregular menstrual cycles.

This evidence suggests the greater the exposure to regular spontaneous menstruation, the greater the likelihood of developing endometriosis. Women now experience over 450 menstruations during their reproductive life, rather than 30–50 that would be expected without contraception and with long periods of lactation as occurred during the last century.

There is now evidence that immune dysfunction is a critical component of the equation, with decreased cytotoxic response to endometrial cells in women with endometriosis due to a defect in natural killer cell activity.

The concentrations of oestrogen and progesterone receptors are lower in endometriotic tissue compared to normal tissue and cyclical variation in endometriotic tissue tends not to occur. Research into the differing growth

Table 3 Examples of sites for endometriotic deposits

Pelvis:
Ovaries may develop endometriotic cyst
Uterosacral ligaments
Pouch of Douglas
Abdominal cavity:
Other peritoneal surfaces
Bowel
Bladder
Umbilicus
Distant sites:
Lungs
Thigh
Vulva

factors present in endometriotic tissue is now an ongoing area of research. The sites for endometriotic deposits can be seen in Table 3.

Diagnosis

History

Patients may be asymptomatic, or have symptoms due to local effects of endometriosis or to complications that have occurred as a result of the disease.

Symptoms include the following:

- *Pain*. Secondary dysmenorrhoea is the classic presentation. Pelvic pain does not correlate well with the total area of endometriosis but does appear to correlate well with the depth of invasion of the lesions. The deeper the infiltration the greater the pelvic pain.
- *Deep dyspareunia*. Intercourse can be painful throughout the menstrual cycle.
- *Infertility*. Historically endometriosis is associated with infertility. However, in the absence of anatomical distortion definitive evidence of a cause–effect relationship has been scanty.
- *Ectopic cyclical bleeding*. This can occur wherever deposits exist and include umbilical, bladder and bowel bleeding.

Examination

Depending on the extent of the disease the examination may reveal nothing significant or may produce clinical findings, including:

- Pelvic mass due to endometrioma.
- Pelvic and abdominal tenderness.
- Tender, thickened uterosacral ligament.
- Fixed retroverted uterus.

Investigation

Unless the deposits are clearly demonstrable on the abdominal wall or vagina, the diagnosis is usually confirmed via the laparoscope.

The extent of the disease can be assessed, with common endometriotic lesions being raised, blue-black nodules just under the peritoneum. A scoring of the extent of the lesions has been developed by the American Fertility Society.

Treatment

Treatment regimes can be directed against the endometriosis itself or directed at the associated symptoms. Asymptomatic patients may require no treatment. Treatment of the infertile patient with minimum disease is controversial as treatment does not improve their chances of conception.

If the patient is symptomatic or has severe disease then medical or surgical treatment or a combination of both can be offered.

Medical treatment

The aim is to prevent the cyclical stimulation of the endometriotic tissue occurring. The general aims are either to produce a pseudo-pregnancy state or a pseudo-menopausal state. Medical treatment is useful in treating pain but 40% of women will get symptoms at some time after treatment stops. Pregnancy rates are not improved with medical treatment.

Drugs used include the following.

Danazol 200–800 mg daily for 6 months. As indicated earlier, danazol suppresses the mid-cycle LH surge and produces a high androgen and low oestrogen environment. The low oestrogen environment does not appear to cause a significant reduction in bone density.

Medroxyprogesterone acetate 30 mg per day for 90 days. This has an endometrial suppression effect and appears effective in producing symptomatic relief.

Gestrinone 2.5 mg twice a week for 90 days. Gestrinone is a synthetic steroid with antigonadotrophic and progestagenic properties. Like medroxyprogesterone acetate it has an endometrial suppression effect and thus appears effective in producing symptomatic relief.

Long-term combined oral contraceptive pill. This produces a pseudo-pregnancy state with regression of endometrial activity.

GnRH agonist. Producing a pseudo-menopausal state by tachyphylaxis, long-acting GnRH agonist given either intranasally or subcutaneously is as effective as danazol or medroxyprogesterone acetate.

Financial implications, as well as the potential effect on bone metabolism, are limiting the use of the agonist. Up to 8% loss of density of the lumbar spine can occur after 6 months' use although this is partially reversible.

Surgical treatment

Disease can either be removed via the laparoscope or via a laparotomy. Normal anatomy can be restored as well as ectopic endometrium being destroyed by laser or diathermy.

The only cure is the resection of all the deposits and hysterectomy with bilateral salpingo-oophorectomy. Hormone replacement therapy is not contraindicated, with a minimal risk of growth of residual endometriosis.

After adequate surgery the recurrence risk is 20%. Fertility can be improved after the treatment of severe disease but this relapses after 1 year post-surgery and then assisted conception techniques should be considered if infertility is the presenting problem.

New developments

Treatment directed against endometriosis in the hope of improving fertility has been disappointing. Research is now being addressed towards treatments that circumvent the implants and attack the symptoms directly. This is directed at immune modulation using the calcium channel blockers verapamil and pentoxifylline. Animal work to date has been encouraging in this area.

Conclusion

With the development of the laparoscope the diagnosis of endometriosis is increasing. Pain is the main indication for treatment, and the disease must be considered as chronic and relapsing rather than an acute phenomenon treatable by a single medical or surgical intervention.

SUGGESTED READING

Shaw, R. W. (ed.) (1990a). *Advances in Reproductive Endocrinology 1. Endometriosis.* Parthenon Publishing Group.
Shaw, R. W. (ed.) (1990b). *Advances in Reproductive Endocrinology 2. Dysfunctional Uterine Bleeding.* Parthenon Publishing Group.
Thomas, E. (1993). Endometriosis. *Br. Med. J.*, **306**, 158–159.

4

Hirsutism, Polycystic Ovarian Syndrome and Amenorrhoea

Michael M. Dooley
West Dorset Hospital, Dorchester, UK

HIRSUTISM

Hirsutism is a common complaint not only in the general practitioner's surgery but also in the gynaecological outpatient department. In the majority of clinical cases the endocrine abnormality is benign and thus it is important to manage the psychological effects of hirsutism.

Definition

Hirsutism is defined as excessive hair growth, with a distribution usually associated with male sexual maturity.

Virilism is defined as masculinisation of the female involving one or more of the following features: clitoral hypertrophy, muscle hypertrophy, breast atrophy, hirsutism and deepening of the voice. Virilism is extremely rare and accounts for less than 1% of patients who are referred with hirsutism.

Pathophysiology

Normal androgen production

In women there is a rapid increase in androgen secretion by the adrenals 2–3 years before menarche (adrenarche).

Understanding Common Disorders in Reproductive Endocrinology. Edited by M.M. Dooley and M.P. Brincat.

Table 1 Factors that influence the levels of SHBG

Increasing levels of SHBG
Pregnancy
Administration of oestrogen
Hyperthyroidism
Decreasing levels of SHBG
Obesity
Hypothyroidism
Administration of danazol

Once ovarian function has reached maturity then both the ovaries and the adrenals are responsible for the secretion of androgens. This can be demonstrated by the decline in the secretion of dehydroepiandrosterone sulphate (DHEAS) after the menopause or after premature ovarian failure.

The most abundant androgens in the normal female are dehydroepiandrosterone (DHEA), DHEAS and androstenedione. These are bound loosely to albumin and are weak androgens.

The more potent androgens are bound to a specific globulin—sex hormone-binding globulin (SHBG)—and these include testosterone, dihydrotestosterone (DHT), androstenediol and the androstenediols.

In the female the concentration of SHBG controls the level of androgen concentration, with no direct control occurring. Bound hormone indicates inactive hormone, with the free hormone being active. Levels of SHBG can be influenced by many factors, and this can be seen in Table 1. Increased levels of SHBG increase the binding of androgens and thus decrease the free, active hormone; the opposite is also true.

The influence of the adrenals on DHEA production is demonstrated by the diurnal variation of DHEA. The influence of the ovaries on testosterone and androstenedione production is demonstrated by the fact that their levels are highest at the midpoint of the menstrual cycle.

Luteinising hormone (LH) and follicle-stimulating hormone (FSH) control ovarian androgen production, which occurs in the theca and ovarian interstitium.

5-α-reductase found in hair follicles and sebaceous glands converts testosterone, androstenedione and DHEA to DHT, the most biologically active androgen. In the female the major source of DHT is androstenedione, produced from both the adrenals and ovaries. Progesterone competes with testosterone for 5 α-reductase and thus this may indicate why anovulation is more often associated with hirsutism.

Oestrone (the major oestrogen in post-menopausal women) is produced by peripheral conversion of androstenedione by the aromatase enzyme, with this occurring in fat and connective tissue.

Pathophysiology in hirsutism

In hirsutism various disorders of androgen physiology can occur, and in most women, with hirsutism, evidence of disturbed androgen production does exist.

Due to the influence of SHBG on testosterone activity simple measurement of total testosterone concentration is a poor guide to altered androgen metabolism.

The majority of idiopathic hirsute patients have been found to have ultrasonographically demonstrable polycystic ovaries (PCO). The ultrasonographic changes are that of a dense echogenic stroma surrounded by a ring of cystic structures 2–5 mm in diameter. These cystic structures can be suppressed by the use of oral contraceptives but the echogenic stroma remains until the menopause.

In these patients increased androgen production, usually by the ovary, is accompanied by reduced SHBG because of obesity and reduced competition with 5 α-reductase due to anovulation. The male sexual hair follicles are then exposed to the increased androgen production.

The fundamental metabolic disturbance in patients with PCO remains unclear although a genetic abnormality is suspected.

Apart from PCO other pathologies that upset androgen production of SHBG binding can lead to hirsutism and these can be seen in Table 2.

Diagnosis

History

Racial and family history gives a clue to a genetic component. Menstrual history may point towards polycystic ovaries. The speed of development of hair growth is important to assess, with rapid growth being associated with a non-benign cause. Symptoms of virilism should also be sought. As certain drugs (phenytoin, diazoxide, glucocorticoids and danazol) may be implicated a good drug history is necessary.

Examination

The following points need to be addressed with regard to the examination:

- Extent of hair growth (NB: enquire about previous local treatment).
- Exclude severe endocrine disease, e.g. acromegaly, Cushing's syndrome.
- Signs of virilism, e.g. cliteromegaly, breast atrophy, male-type baldness.

Table 2 Causes of hirsutism

Genetic	Racial Familial (? associated with PCO)[9]
Physiological	Puberty Pregnancy Menopause
Endocrine (non-androgen-producing)	Hypothyroidism Acromegaly
Androgen excess	
Ovarian causes	Polycystic ovaries Gonadal dysgenesis Tumours Arrhenoblastomas Lipoid cell tumours Hilus cell tumours
Adrenal	Congenital adrenal hyperplasia Adrenal adenoma/carcinoma Cushing's syndrome
Congenital	Hurler's syndrome De Lange's syndrome
Porphyria	
Hamartomas	
Drugs	Phenytoin Diazoxide Glucocorticoids Danazol
CNS lesions	Multiple sclerosis Encephalitis

Investigations

At the initial visit the following investigations should be arranged:

1. *Serum testosterone level.* Normal or slightly elevated level will suggest a benign cause. High level suggests an androgen-secreting tumour.
2. *Serum DHEA and androstenedione.* Raised levels indicate an adrenal origin of the excess androgens.
3. *Serum 17β-hydroxyprogesterone.* Raised levels indicate congenital adrenal hyperplasia.
4. *Serum SHBG.* A low level of SHBG is associated with a raised total testosterone level and a high free testosterone level.
5. *Serum LH and FSH concentrations.* A raised LH/FSH ratio is consistent with polycystic ovarian disease.

6. *Serum thyroxine levels.* Hypothyroidism is associated with hirsutism.
7. *Ovarian ultrasonography.* This is used to detect PCO and other ovarian tumours.

After the above investigations are completed investigations for specific endocrine disorders should be performed when indicated. For example, if 17β-hydroxyprogesterone levels are elevated an adrenocorticotrophic hormone (ACTH) stimulation test should be performed.

Treatment

Treatment needs to include full and adequate explanation; the majority of women have a benign condition that may require significant psychological support. Serious conditions, if diagnosed, need to be treated appropriately.

Local treatment

This may be the most effective and does not stimulate further growth. Bleaching agents, waxes, depilatory creams and shaving all have a role.

Specific treatment

This is directed at the suppression of androgen production from the adrenal and the ovary as well as the use of specific antiandrogens. It is important to emphasise that therapy is lengthy (12–24 months) and immediate improvement should not be expected.

Such methods of specific treatment include the following:

- *Ovarian suppression.* This can be achieved by the use of the combined oral contraceptive pill. The progestagen inhibits LH secretion, which results in reduction of ovarian androgen production. The oestrogen increases SHBG levels, thus increasing testosterone binding and reducing testosterone activity. Oestrogens also reduce 5α-reductase levels in the skin, resulting in reduced conversion to DHT. Oral contraceptives containing levonorgestrel should be avoided as this is a testosterone derivative.
- *Adrenal suppression.* This is achieved by glucocorticoids but should only be used in women with proven adrenal causes, e.g. congenital adrenal hyperplasia. Low doses of dexamethasone (0.25–1.0 mg nocte) have been used, with some beneficial effect.
- *Antiandrogens.* These are substances that prevent androgens from exerting their activity in the target tissues at the intracellular receptor.

Cyproterone acetate (CPA) and spironolactone have been used in gynaecology and recently cimetidine has been investigated. CPA is a steroid derived from 17β-hydroxyprogesterone and has antiandrogen, progestational and antigonadotrophic actions. It is administered orally in a reverse sequential regime in which CPA 100 mg per day is given on days 5–15 of the menstrual cycle and ethinyloestradiol 30 μg per day is given on days 5–26 of the cycle.

This combination therapy reduces plasma testosterone and androstenedione levels, suppresses gonadotrophins and increases SHBG. It also provides good cycle control and contraception. Reduction of CPA can occur down to a maintenance level of 2 mg per day.

Spironolactone is an aldosterone antagonist that is a potent antiandrogen, binding to the androgen receptor in the hair follicle. Side-effects include menstrual irregularity and menorrhagia. Treatment with spironolactone should be started at a dose of 50 mg per day on days 4–21 of the cycle or, preferably, continuously with a combined oral contraceptive.

Conclusion

A patient presenting with hirsutism needs sympathy and understanding. Appropriate investigations need to be performed to exclude a rare sinister cause, especially if virilism is present. In idiopathic hirsutism, local treatment will give immediate relief but therapeutic agents will take 12–24 months to have an effect.

POLYCYSTIC OVARIAN SYNDROME

In 1935 Stein and Leventhal described a syndrome of anovulation, hirsutism and obesity associated with enlarged and polycystic ovaries. Initially described as Stein–Leventhal syndrome, this condition has now been termed polycystic ovarian syndrome (PCOS).

With the development of transabdominal and transvaginal ultrasound, a reliable non-invasive method of diagnosis is available. With these advanced diagnostic facilities PCOS has proved to be not only common but also quite heterogeneous.

Pathophysiology

PCOS is a disorder of multisystem involvement representing hypothalamic–pituitary–ovarian/adrenal interaction.

Chronic stimulation by LH, compounded by hyperinsulinaemia, combined with the overall increased amount of androgen secretory stromal and thecal tissue present in the ovary are major reasons for the excessive rate of ovarian androgen secretion in PCOS.

Ovarian rates of aromatisable and non-aromatisable androgen secretion are enhanced in PCOS. This may be due to LH-stimulated increases in androgen synthesis with the thecae of individual follicles or to a net increase in the overall number of androgen secretory atretic follicles which accumulate. The increased rate of follicular atresia causes a build-up of secondary interstitial tissue in the ovarian stroma (hyperthecosis), which is a major site of excessive androgen synthesis in PCO.

There is a quantitative deficiency of circulating FSH leading to anovulation.

Fasting insulin concentrations are raised in one third of lean and 75% of obese women with PCOS. Insulin and possibly insulin-like growth factor 1 has a gonadotrophin action promoting ovarian androgen synthesis and thus contributing to menstrual disturbance. This effect of insulin on the ovary may account for the fact that obesity causes for a greater expression of PCOS and why dietary advice is a valuable approach to treatment.

Diagnosis

Diagnostic criteria have remained controversial. Diagnosis may be on a combination of oligomenorrhoea and elevated androgen concentration, or more strict criteria including ultrasonographic diagnosis in combination with hirsutism, oligomenorrhoea and elevated serum androgen and LH concentrations. In Table 3 are some general guidelines that facilitate diagnosis.

Treatment

Treatment depends on the presenting feature. Hirsutism was dealt with earlier in this chapter. A summary of different treatment approaches can be seen in Table 4.

Infertility

Spontaneous ovulation can occur in PCOS, but if the patient is anovulatory first-line treatment is with an antioestrogen such as clomiphene citrate. Ovulation rates are high and in those who respond satisfactorily conception rates are near normal. Adjuvant treatment with pre-treatment progesterone or timed human chorionic gonadotrophin (HCG) may be useful. Miscarriage rates are increased and this may be associated with the elevation in background LH.

Table 3 Useful indicators in the diagnosis of polycystic ovaries

History	Anovulatory dysfunctional uterine bleeding Oligomenorrhoea or amenorrhoea Hirsutism Obesity (not always) Infertility Possible family history Recurrent miscarriage associated with increased LH
Examination	Obese Hirsute Palpable ovaries
Investigations	Ultrasound Enlarged ovaries Dense echogenic stroma Ring of 2–5 mm cystic structures Elevated testosterone Elevated LH/FSH ratio Elevated androstenedione 17β-Hydroxyprogesterone } may be elevated Prolactin } may be elevated SHBG may be reduced May have insulin resistance

Table 4 Available treatment regimes for patients with PCOS

Problem	Treatment
General	Explanation and reassurance
Infertility (due to anovulation)	Clomiphene citrate Gonadotrophins LHRH analogue + gonadotrophins Laparoscopic ovarian surgery
Recurrent miscarriage	LHRH analogue + gonadotrophins
Hirsutism	Local treatment Specific treatment Ovarian suppression: oral contraceptive Adrenal suppression: dexamethasone Antiandrogens Cyproterone acetate Spironolactone Cimetidine
Obesity	Weight reduction
Menstrual irregularities	Oral contraceptives Hormone replacement therapy Progestagens

Gonadotrophin stimulation therapy has been conventionally accepted as first-line treatment for infertile women with PCOS who fail to conceive in response to administration of clomiphene citrate.

Pure FSH may be used in preference to human menopausal gonadotrophin in order to prevent further LH stimulation.

Careful monitoring of treatment cycles is essential to avoid multiple pregnancy and ovarian hyperstimulation syndrome. This can be performed using ultrasonography and also oestrogen monitoring. Conception rates are of the order of 30–40%.

Pre-HCG luteinisation is another problem with this treatment. This is caused by a surge or rise in endogenous LH in response to increasing plasma oestradiol concentrations before the criteria for administration of the ovulatory dose of HCG are achieved.

To prevent the problems of pre-HCG luteinisation a combined therapy has been developed using the antigonadotrophic effects of luteinising hormone-releasing hormone analogue when used in a tachyphylactic mode to suppress endogenous pituitary LH activity during simultaneous induction of follicular growth and ovulation using exogenous gonadotrophins. Pregnancy rates using this regime are of the order of 35% in the first cycle and 80% cumulative over 6 months.

Treatment of clomiphene-resistant anovulation by laparoscopic ovarian surgery with multiple punch resection, laser vaporisation and ovarian electrocautery has recently gained attention. Post-operatively there is a rapid decrease in testosterone and androstenedione levels, whereas LH levels decline more slowly until the first menstrual period. A significant increase in FSH has also been demonstrated. It is possible that 'damage' to the ovary produces a change in the intra-ovarian androgenic milieu leading to restoration of the cycle.

Recurrent miscarriages

Elevated levels of LH leading to a hyperandrogenic environment within the follicle and premature ageing of the oocyte are suggested factors contributing to subfertility and poor pregnancy outcome in patients with PCOS. The increased incidence of miscarriage with PCOS could theoretically be reduced by the inhibition of LH hypersecretion. Studies to date are few but findings do suggest that pituitary suppression is a promising method for treating PCOS patients with recurrent abortions and possibly with unexplained infertility.

Hirsutism

This has been fully discussed earlier in the chapter and a summary is given in Table 4.

Obesity

Weight reduction is indicated and by the effect on insulin, androgen and oestrogen levels the clinical effects of PCO may be greatly reduced.

Oligomenorrhoea and amenorrhoea

If infertility is a problem the appropriate treatment regime needs to be followed. If it is not a problem then it is important to address the risk of osteoporosis in these women. Although the raised androgens may help protect against osteoporosis the general opinion is that oestrogen replacement therapy needs to be given. This can be in the form of the combined oral contraceptive pill or standard hormone replacement therapy, although the latter will not provide contraceptive cover.

Some anovulatory women will develop endometrial hyperplasia due to unopposed oestrogen stimulation, and although progestagen treatment will help prevent this long-term oestrogen combination therapy is perhaps more beneficial, with better patient compliance.

AMENORRHOEA

Definition

Primary amenorrhoea

This is defined as: no menstruation by 14 years of age with growth failure or absence of secondary sexual characteristics, i.e. breast development and pubic hair growth; or no menstruation by 16 years of age when growth and sexual development are normal. (Primary amenorrhoea is discussed in Chapter 2.)

Secondary amenorrhoea

This is defined as absence of menses for 6 months in a previously menstruating woman.

Incidence

Amenorrhoea occurs in 10–20% of patients complaining of subfertility and is a common reason for referral to a gynaecology clinic.

Table 5 Classification of secondary amenorrhoea

Physiological	Pregnancy Menopause
Primary ovarian failure	Premature menopause Resistant ovarian syndrome
Gonadotrophin abnormality	Hyperprolactinaemia Structural problems in pituitary or hypothalamus, e.g. craniopharyngioma Hypogonadotrophic hypogonadisms, e.g. Kallman's syndrome PCOS Weight loss Chronic illness Psychogenic
Genital tract abnormality	Ashermann's syndrome
Other endocrinopathies	Thyroid dysfunction

Aetiology

Amenorrhoea is a symptom, not a disease, and has a variety of causes (see Table 5). There is an overlap between primary and secondary amenorrhoea.

Secondary problems associated with amenorrhoea

Osteoporosis

Women who are amenorrhoeic run a significant risk of oestrogen deficiency. Osteoporosis is now well demonstrated in this group, with up to 10% bone loss occurring over 1 year.

Other hypo-oestrogenic complications

These include dyspareunia, depression and decreased libido.

Endometrial hyperplasia

This can occur if unopposed oestrogen is produced. It usually presents with oligomenorrhoea although it can be associated (although rarely) with amenorrhoea.

Hirsutism

As a result of reduction in progesterone secretion hirsutism can develop. This is due to the evidence that progesterone and testosterone compete for the enzyme 5α-reductase. If there is no luteal phase then a greater proportion of testosterone is converted to the biologically more active DHT.

Diagnosis of secondary amenorrhoea

History

It is important to take a full history. Hyperprolactinaemia will be suspected if there is a history of galactorrhoea. A space-occupying lesion within the pituitary may cause headaches and visual disturbances. Hyperprolactinaemia can be due to drug therapy and such drugs include neuroleptics, antidepressants, antihistamines, antihypertensives, antiemetics and opiates.

Stress, vigorous exercise and weight changes (either increase or decrease) can be associated with amenorrhoea and are thus important to detect.

Hirsutism and acne may be associated with PCOS although if associated with other virilising symptoms the cause may be more sinister, including a virilising tumour of the ovary.

Recent gynaecological surgery, especially post-partum evacuation for retained products of conception, may indicate Ashermann's syndrome with the development of intrauterine adhesions. If the patient at the same time complains of pre-menstrual syndrome-like symptoms then further suspicion of this diagnosis is raised.

The secondary effects of hypo-oestrogenism need to be assessed, including dry vagina, hot flushes and night sweats.

Loss of smell may be associated with Kallman's syndrome.

Examination

A full examination needs to be done. Specific attention needs to be addressed to body mass index, which is the weight in kilograms divided by the square of the height in metres (BMI = kg/m^2), the normal range being between 20 and 25.

Gross changes due to endocrinopathies need to be determined, including thyroid disease and Cushing's syndrome.

Evidence of hirsutism, acne and other signs of virilisation need to be addressed.

Investigation

Radiological

Ultrasound. A most important advance in the ability to investigate a patient with menstrual disturbances is the development of high-resolution ultrasound. The ultrasonic assessment of uterine size is useful in primary amenorrhoea, a pre-pubertal uterus having a different shape and cervical length from a fully stimulated one.

Endometrial development can be assessed over time and is an ideal end organ bioassay for oestrogen.

Ovarian ultrasonic assessment has already been fully discussed in the section on polycystic ovaries.

Computed tomography and magnetic resonance imaging. Computed tomographic scan or magnetic resonance imaging of the pituitary is useful to assess if an adenoma is present when the prolactin levels are raised.

Blood investigation

Prolactin. Under normal conditions serum prolactin levels are highest in the early morning and may be influenced by meals, exercise and sexual activity. For diagnostic purposes the optimal time is to obtain levels in late morning, with fasting and abstinence from exercise or sexual activity.

Gonadotrophin levels. FSH will be raised (>20 IU/1) in cases of primary ovarian failure. The LH/FSH ratio may be raised in PCOS. Subnormal LH and FSH with low oestradiol indicates hypogonadotrophic hypogonadism.

Thyroid function. Hypothyroidism can lead to amenorrhoea and cause an elevation in prolactin levels.

Serum oestradiol levels. These may be helpful in certain cases (e.g. premature ovarian failure) when the levels will be low.

Androgens (NB: testosterone and androstenedione) and SHBG. These are useful if there is a suspicion of PCOS.

Karyotype. Turner's syndrome (X0) is associated with premature ovarian failure and this usually occurs when a mosaic pattern is present.

Dynamic investigations

Progestagen withdrawal bleed. Progestagen causes withdrawal bleed on an oestrogen-primed endometrium. If a progestagen challenge is given (e.g. medroxyprogesterone acetate 5 mg b.d. × 10 days) and a withdrawal bleed occurs this indicates oestrogen stimulation of the endometrium, and the diagnosis is usually anovulation.

Treatment

Management of patients with amenorrhoea should be directed at treating the underlying disorder, e.g. weight loss. Thyroid disease needs to be treated appropriately. Sometimes reassurance and time is all that is required.

Ovarian failure in itself cannot be treated but hormone replacement therapy is needed to prevent secondary pathology, including osteoporosis.

Ashermann's syndrome can sometimes be corrected by hysteroscopic removal of adhesions, although conception rarely occurs.

If the patient with hypogonadotrophic hypogonadism requests return of fertility then human menopausal gonadotrophin (HMG) is indicated, with HCG being used to cause ovum release mid-cycle.

For hyperprolactinaemia, surgery remains effective treatment. However, the role is currently extremely limited. Dopamine agonists (e.g. bromocriptine) have now become the primary modality used to treat micro- and macroadenomas of the pituitary. Bromocriptine is an ergot derivative that is metabolised in the liver and acts by decreasing the secretion and synthesis of prolactin by the lactotrophs and also causes a reduction in the cytoplasmic volume of the lactotrophs.

Normal doses of bromocriptine is 2.5 mg orally up to three times a day; 70–80% of patients with hyperprolactinaemia respond with decreasing prolactin levels and the resolution of symptoms. The side-effects are noted in Table 6.

Tumour shrinkage is evident in most patients and macroadenomas respond in a similar way to microadenomas except it may take longer for the levels to normalise. Although there is no evidence that bromocriptine is teratogenic or that there is an increased fetal wastage, therapy should be discontinued during pregnancy. Only 1% of microadenomas progress during pregnancy but macroadenomas have a greater propensity to expand. Patients with macroadenomas need to be carefully monitored and treatment

Table 6 Side-effects with bromocriptine

Gastrointestinal	Nausea Vomiting
Cardiovascular	Dizziness Syncope
Less common side-effects	Headache Nasal congestion Abdominal cramps Constipation
High-dose complications	Hallucinations Confusion Seizures

should be re-initiated after the onset of symptoms such as headache or visual field loss.

When bromocriptine treatment is discontinued growth of the tumour mass generally recurs, although prolonged treatment may cause permanent tissue death.

Conclusion

Amenorrhoea is a common symptom associated with conditions including osteoporosis and infertility. Appropriate investigations allow for timely management and the prevention of long-term, potentially serious sequelae.

SUGGESTED READING

Philosophe, R. and Seibel, M. (1991). Novel approaches to the management of hyperprolactinaemia. *Curr. Opinion Obstet. Gynaecol.*, **3**, 336–342.

Ruutiainen, K. and Seppala, M. (1991). Polycystic ovary syndrome: evolution of a concept. *Curr. Opinion Obstet. Gynaecol.*, **3**, 326–335.

Shaw, R. W. (ed.) (1991). *Advances in Reproductive Endocrinology 3. Polycystic Ovaries.* Parthenon Publishing.

5
Infertility

Marc Formosa and Mark P. Brincat
St. Luke's Hospital Medical School, Malta

Infertility is a common problem affecting one in six couples wishing to conceive. A structured approach to investigation and treatment is essential. Psychological effects of infertility can compound an already stressful situation. Early referral to a specialist centre is important if pregnancy is not achieved relatively quickly.

Much of the improvement that has taken place in the investigation and diagnosis of couples has not been paralleled by improvements in pregnancy rates. The management of infertility therefore remains a time-consuming, often costly exercise that can end in further frustration to both patients and doctor.

Infertility is best defined as the inability to conceive after 1 year of unprotected intercourse. Changes in lifestyle, family structure and particularly in the female role have led to a greater proportion of women postponing childbearing to the later reproductive years.

As a rule one would avoid an aggressive approach to infertility before 3 years (e.g. *in vitro* fertilisation (IVF)) but if the woman is 35 years or older this may be considered earlier.

About 10–15% of couples have been estimated to be infertile, which represents about one in 10 of new referrals to a general gynaecological clinic.

The increased incidence of infertility with age is shown in Table 1.

Infertility is more common in Negro populations when compared to white—18.1% versus 9.4%—the difference being mainly due to an increased incidence of tubal disease.

Infertility decreases with increasing parity up to parity three and then it increases slightly (Table 2).

Understanding Common Disorders in Reproductive Endocrinology. Edited by M.M. Dooley and M.P. Brincat.

Table 1 Infertility with age

Age (years)	Percentage incidence of infertility
15–19	2.1%
20–24	6.4%
36–39	12.5%
40–44	15.9%

Table 2 Infertility versus parity

Para 0	18.1%
Para 1	12.4%
Para 2	6.0%
Para >3	7.9%

After the first year of unprotected intercourse 75% of normal couples would have achieved a pregnancy, while after 2 years the figure is 90%.

Infertility can be differentiated into primary (no previous pregnancies) and secondary (previous pregnancies). This is only useful in that the incidence of causes for each are different, e.g. secondary infertility is more likely to be due to tubal damage, while male factors are more likely in primary infertility.

AETIOLOGY

The main causes of infertility can be seen in Table 3.

Table 3 Causes of infertility

Ovulatory failure	20%
Tubal damage	15%
Endometriosis	5%
Mucus defect	5%
Sperm defects	25%
Other male problems	2%
Coital failure	2%
Unexplained	30%
Others	10%

NB: Some couples may have more than one cause.

SCHEME OF INVESTIGATION OF INFERTILITY

The basic essentials are:

1. Full history and examination of both partners, including a detailed coital history.
2. Ovulation assessment.
3. Semen microscopy.
4. Sperm–mucus penetration.
5. Tubal assessment, usually via laparoscope.
6. Appropriate use of hysteroscope and hysterosalpingogram.

History of the female

The first factor to consider is the age of the patient: at 35 years the chance of conception is half that at age 25, while at 40 they diminish further to one fifth (20%).

The duration of infertility and the age of the patient will indicate the pace with which investigation proceeds and what therapeutic approach is to be offered.

Menstrual history—rarely does a woman have a 28-day cycle, but the regularity is as important as the cycle length. It is more worrying if the cycle is short rather than if it is long. (NB: oligomenorrhoea is defined as a cycle longer than 42 days.)

The presence of dysmenorrhoea must be classified. Primary dysmenorrhoea is defined as pain beginning on the first day of menstruation and as menstruation proceeds the pain improves. It is usually associated with ovulation. Secondary dysmenorrhoea is pain beginning 1–5 days prior to the onset of menstruation and is relieved by menstruation. The latter is considered to be related to pelvic disease, e.g. endometriosis, fibroids and pelvic inflammatory disease. Mid-cycle pain and vaginal discharge may be biological markers of ovulation. Only 30% of patients will admit to recognising ovulation at the initial visit.

The method of contraception previously adopted by the patient may be associated with infertility. This is especially so for intrauterine contraceptive devices (IUCD). The pill is not a cause of infertility. Pill takers have lower pregnancy rates in the first 3 months after stopping the pill but by 1 year pregnancy rates similar to those in people coming off natural forms of contraception are achieved.

Galactorrhoea is uncommon; although hyperprolactinaemia is a frequent cause of infertility (about 5%), only 30% of patients with high prolactin levels will also have galactorrhoea.

The past obstetric history, including any spontaneous or therapeutic termination of pregnancy, ectopic gestations and complications of any deliveries, are particularly relevant to infertility.

The occupation of the patient and other aspects of her lifestyle will provide information regarding risk factors for infertility, e.g. pelvic inflammatory disease.

Frequency of sexual intercourse must be determined, this being usually related to age. At age 20 years a frequency of five times a week is average, while at 40 years this would be closer to once a week. It is not uncommon, however, to receive false information regarding the frequency of sexual relations. Since conceptions occur through a 3-day window, a frequency of intercourse of four times a week does not bind conception strictly to day 14. The presence of dyspareunia may indicate the presence of pelvic disease or it may simply be positional; it may also be a complaint used to mask deeper sexual problems.

The male partner should be asked whether there is any difficulty maintaining an erection, whether there is any premature ejaculation and whether penetration occurs properly.

Any past endocrine abnormality or pelvic surgery of any type must be recorded in detail. Vaginal surgery is also important, for example a cone biopsy. This may restrict the production of cervical mucus and sperm transport cannot occur properly. This may also follow laser ablation or large loop excision of the cervix.

As previously stated, the social and occupational history of the patient is important. Smoking more than 10 cigarettes a day will interfere with tubal function. Nicotine interferes with cilial action in the tube as it does with that in the chest.

Examination of the female

A basic general examination with particular attention to height and weight, body hair, thyroid and breasts is important. A low body mass index is associated with subfertility. Body mass index is calculated by dividing the weight in kilograms by the height in metres squared (BMI = kg/m^2).

The presence of galactorrhoea should be demonstrated. A thorough gynaecological examination is mandatory, with due care being given to the appearance of the external genitalia. A cervical smear, if indicated, is taken.

Any suspicion of abnormality of the genitalia or Müllerian tube defects should be excluded by appropriate investigations, i.e. karyotyping if intersex is suspected or hysterosalpingogram/laparoscopy if Müllerian tube agenesis is suspected.

History of the male

It is estimated that in approximately 30% of infertile couples the cause lies partially or wholly with the male.

The age of the patient is not as important as in the female; normal sperm counts can be maintained up to 50–60 years. A history of a past pregnancy with another partner confirms fertilisation capacity. Exposure to radiation (X-rays), a hot environment, chemicals or drugs (e.g. Salazopyrin) must be excluded. A full alcohol and smoking history is also important.

Long stressful hours may suggest a low frequency of intercourse. A past history of inguinal hernia repairs, testicular tumours or orchidopexy and any chemotherapy must be sought.

Past urinary tract or genital infection, especially mumps orchitis, is recorded.

Examination of the male

Examination should be performed to ensure that genitalia are normal. The size and consistency of the testicles should be noted as well as the presence of vasa deferentia and varicocele.

Investigations of the female

Assessment of ovarian activity

Changes in cervical mucus. Pre-ovulatory cervical mucus is plentiful, clear, acellular and with a low viscosity. Spinnbarkeit can be demonstrated and cervical mucus in the pre-ovulatory phase ferns on drying. On the day of ovulation threads as long as 15–20 cm can be formed without breaking. The cervical os opens slightly at the time of ovulation.

Endometrial biopsy. The presence of secretory endometrium simply confirms the presence of progesterone but is not confirmatory for ovulation, e.g. luteinised unruptured follicle (LUF cycle).

Basal body temperature. On average a patient gets bored with keeping a basal body temperature chart after 2 months and this may also compound the stressful situation of infertility. Mistakes in charting are common. This method identifies a shift in temperature which points out when progesterone is produced rather than when ovulation occurs. It does, however, give an idea of the length of the luteal phase. In the light of available evidence the role of basal body temperature recording is now reducing significantly.

Laparoscopy. This needs to be done in the luteal phase in order to confirm ovulation, but if performed in the follicular phase the developing follicle should be identified.

Ultrasound. Sequential ultrasound examination will demonstrate growth of the dominant follicle and in addition to oestradiol and luteinising hormone (LH) levels will confirm whether growth is appropriate.

A rising LH level is a sensitive indication of ovulation but in the case of the luteinised unruptured follicle a rise will still occur.

Hormone levels. Assessment of reproductive hormones—follicle stimulating hormone (FSH), luteinising hormone (LH) and prolactin in the early follicular phase, and progesterone in the mid-luteal phase—is an important part of the diagnosis work-up of infertility.

If the periods follow a normal regular cycle then a prolactin level is not essential. See Chapter 4 for further details on amenorrhoea and polycystic ovarian syndrome (PCOS).

Testosterone and androstenedione levels are useful in the diagnosis of PCOS.

Tubal patency

Laparoscopic examination with dye insertion. This allows assessment of the pelvic anatomy and any pathology including adhesions, endometriosis, ovarian disease and tubal patency.

Hysterosalpingogram (HSG). HSG demonstrates intrauterine and tubal anatomy as well as patency. It provides no further information with regard to pelvic anatomy.

Hysteroscopy

This can allow detailed investigations of the uterine cavity and treatment if appropriate.

Rubella status

Rubella status should be checked before commencing any treatment.

General investigations

If indicated, general investigations may include a full blood count, thyroid function test and random glucose.

Cervical factors

The investigation of cervical factors as a cause of infertility can be by the following methods:

1. Post-coital test (PCT).
2. Crossed hostility test.
3. Antisperm antibodies.

The PCT involves the aspiration of a sample of cervical mucus around the time of ovulation (detected either by ultrasound examination or urinary LH surge detection) within 6 hours of intercourse.

The World Health Organization definition of a positive PCT is when 15 or more active sperm per high-powered field are present. It is negative if there are five or less.

If there are no sperm at all, not even dead ones, one should suspect that no normal sexual intercourse took place. A negative test is of limited value as it may indicate poor timing and/or an infection as well as mucus hostility.

A crossed hostility test or formal sperm penetration test should be performed in the event of a negative PCT.

Methods of performing a crossed hostility test. The couple are advised to avoid sexual intercourse for 3 days and after that a separate sample of the male's semen and female's mucus are obtained. These are tested separately in the following combinations:

1. Male versus female.
2. Male versus fertile donor (mucus).
3. Male fertile donor sperm versus female's mucus.
4. Fertile male donor sperm versus fertile female donor mucus.

In a local hospital setting a sperm/mucus challenge is enough. The preparation is observed over a 20 min period and the formation of phalenx as the sperm ascends through the mucus is to be regarded as normal.

Where this test is abnormal antisperm antibodies should be sought in both serum and semen samples. A full understanding of antisperm antibodies has not yet been developed. Cervical factors are responsible for about 3% of cases of infertility.

Investigations of the male

Semen analysis. This should be collected after a minimum of 3 days' abstinence and a maximum of 5 days. The sample should be in the laboratory within 1 h of production. The results for a normal sample are shown in Table 4.

Table 4 Normal semen parameters

Volume 2–6 ml, liquefaction within 30 min
Density > 20 × 10^6/ml
Motility > 40% forward progression after 2 h
Morphology > 40% normal
White blood cells < 1 × 10^6/ml
A minimum of two samples needs to be assessed

Hormone investigations. If azoospermia is present then serum LH, FSH, testosterone and prolactin levels should be performed on the male. If the FSH is high, chromosomal analysis to check for Klinefelter's syndrome is performed.

Urine analysis. Aspermia may represent impotence requiring psychological help, or retrograde ejaculation requiring a post-coital urine assessment.

Culture of sperm. Oligospermia may be associated with infection, and culture needs to be performed.

Antisperm antibodies. Sperm-agglutinating or immobilising antibodies have been estimated to occur in 3–13% of infertile males.

Agglutination. Spontaneous agglutination indicates that there are sperm-agglutinating antibodies in the seminal fluid or that the sperm is infected.

TREATMENT

General

It is important not to convert a problem into an obsession by unnecessary investigations, anecdotal evidence and unrealistic expectations.

Counselling is very important and a trained counsellor should be available when indicated. The Human Fertilisation and Embryology Act 1990 established access to proper counselling as mandatory.

Psychosexual help should also be available if indicated and psychosexual problems should be highlighted in the history.

General advice should be given about the avoidance of alcohol and smoking.

It is important to give the couple realistic expectations of the results, and Figure 1 gives the cumulative conception rates of treated cycles.

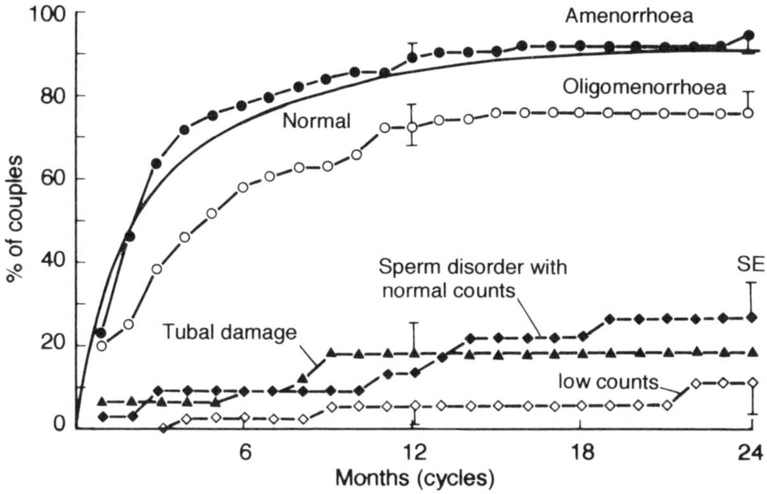

Figure 1 Cumulative conception rates of the most and least successfully treated of the common causes of infertility, compared with normal, excluding the use of donor insemination, or IVF, or surgery for reversal of sterilisation. (SE = standard error, which is a statistical guide to the confidence limits of a graph.) Reproduced from *British Medical Journal* 1985, **21**, 1693, with permission

Treatment of sperm disorders

Sperm disorders are the single most common cause of subfertility. There are limited treatment regimes, which include the following.

Artificial insemination. Artificial insemination with the partner's sperm, whether prepared or fresh, has now been shown to be of no benefit.

Superovulation with intrauterine insemination. Superovulation with intrauterine insemination is helpful for unexplained infertility with multiple recruitment of oocytes. It has a limited role with sperm disorder problems. It does, however, carry a risk of multiple pregnancy, and ultrasound monitoring of the number of follicles needs to be carried out before insemination.

In vitro fertilisation (IVF). IVF is now playing a greater role in male factor problems and is expanded later and in Chapter 6.

Microinjection techniques. Microinjection techniques for IVF are being explored for the most severe cases.

Donor insemination (DI). Great care in counselling the couple needs to be taken before embarking on this course of therapy. DI should only be carried out in centres where sperm banks exist. Donors need to be carefully screened and, in accordance with current recommendations, frozen sperm only used. The advent of human immunodeficiency virus (HIV) risk has made the use of fresh sperm contraindicated. Unfortunately this has led to a lower pregnancy rate since frozen sperm results consistently fail to be as good as results with fresh sperm.

Donor insemination in the UK is regulated by the Human Fertilisation and Embryology Authority (HFEA).

The HFEA is a statutory body that was established in the UK after the passage of the Human Fertilisation and Embryology Act in 1990. The body inspects and licenses centres with the provision of being able to bring the full weight of the criminal law to bear for serious offences. Without a licence, no one can create an embryo (including an egg in the process of fertilisation), keep or use an embryo, store gametes, or in the course of providing treatment service to any woman use donated sperm or donated eggs or mix gametes with the live gametes of other animals.

Treatment of disorders of ovulation

Given accurate diagnosis, all women except those with premature menopause can be very effectively treated, as shown in Figure 2.

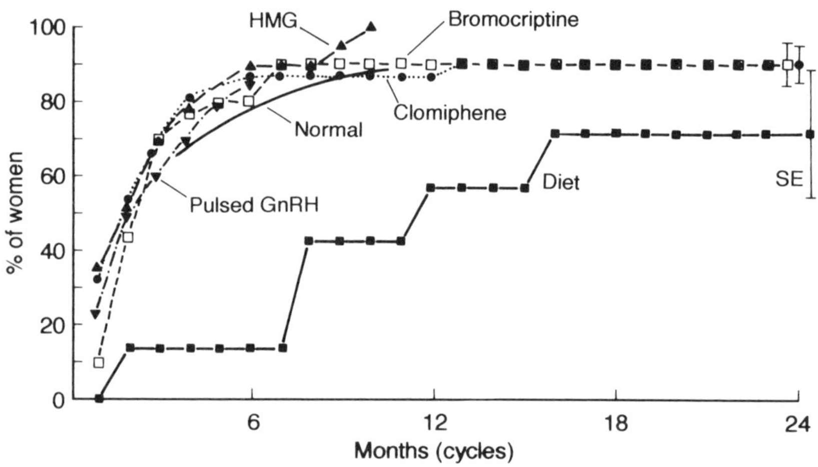

Figure 2 Cumulative conception rates resulting from individual treatment methods as appropriate in women with amenorrhoea, compared with normal. GnRH = gonadotrophine-releasing hormone, given using a portable battery-driven pump. HMG = human menopausal gonadotrophins, given as a daily injection. Clomiphene and bromocriptine are taken as tablets. Reproduced from *British Medical Journal* 1985, **21**, 1693, with permission

Ovarian failure

This may be either primary, presenting with primary amenorrhoea, or secondary, presenting with secondary amenorrhoea. The condition is associated with universally unsuccessful conventional treatment and the only option remaining is oocyte donation, which is proven to be very successful, with pregnancy rates of the order of 40% per cycle.

Polycystic ovarian syndrome

This condition, previously known as Stein–Leventhal syndrome, is characterised by oligomenorrhoea (cycles longer than 42 days), obesity and hirsutism.

Hormone analysis will reveal a raised LH/FSH ratio of the order of 3:1. Care must be taken in menstruating women to take the serum sample in the early follicular phase as LH in the luteal phase may be down-regulated if progesterone is present.

The pulsatile secretion of FSH and LH is abnormal in PCOS. The high level of LH can interfere with chromosome division from metaphase I to metaphase II at the time of ovulation. If the ovum is not released in metaphase II then the ova are not suitable for ovulation. This accounts for a high percentage of spontaneous abortion in PCOS patients.

For a full discussion on PCOS refer to Chapter 4.

Anovulatory infertility

Clomiphene citrate. This compound is oestrogenic and antioestrogenic at the same time. It should not be given to patients who are ovulating because it will interfere with oestradiol receptors in the endometrium, raise basal LH levels and affect the production of cervical mucus.

Clomiphene should be started in a dose of 50 mg for 5 days from day 2 to day 6 of the cycle. The serum progesterone should be assessed in the mid-luteal phase and if no ovulation occurs the dose is raised to 100 mg and then to 150 mg. There is, however, no benefit in going above that level.

As long as no other abnormality exists treatment should continue for at least 9–12 months unless the patient conceives.

If ovulation does not occur at a dose of 150 mg, follicular growth should be monitored by ultrasound scanning in the next cycle and oestradiol checked on days 10 and 13 and progesterone on day 21.

If the oestradiol rise is consistent with the presence of a follicle but a low level of progesterone then luteinisation may not be occurring. In the absence of an LH surge, human chorionic gonadotrophin (HCG) can be given along with clomiphene. If both oestradiol and progesterone are flat then gonadotrophins should be considered. Human menopausal gonadotrophin (HMG) or pure FSH therapy must, however, have good monitoring with ultrasound and possibly hormonal assays.

Gonadotrophins. HMG is a mixture of FSH/LH, having mainly an action of FSH, i.e. follicular growth. Ovum release and luteinisation can be achieved by using HCG.

The regime for HMG is to give a dose of 150 IU by intramuscular injection on days 1, 3, 5, etc., to stimulate follicular growth.

Other regimes include daily administration with or without clomiphene citrate. A pure FSH preparation may also be used, especially in cases of PCOS.

When the follicular response is adequate, i.e. no more than three follicles greater than 18 mm diameter as detected by ultrasound scanning, HCG may be given and the couple advised to have sexual intercourse.

Monitoring with oestradiol levels only will not indicate the degree of follicular development, i.e. two small follicles will produce as much oestradiol as one large one. It is best to monitor with a combination of oestradiol levels and ultrasound examination. The main complication to be avoided with this treatment is ovarian hyperstimulation syndrome (OHSS).

OHSS is a complication of induction of ovulation in which there is excessive stimulation of the ovaries. It usually occurs after HCG has been given. Other risk factors include younger age, women with PCOS and previous history of OHSS. Early pregnancy is also a predisposing factor due to HCG ovarian stimulation.

Mild OHSS refers to enlargement of the ovaries with cyst formation. The patient complains of abdominal discomfort and heaviness, swelling and pain. Treatment is conservative, with simple analgesics if required.

Moderate OHSS develops when the pain is more severe and the ovarian cysts enlarged. Nausea, vomiting and diarrhoea are present and there is some weight gain. Close observation is needed to monitor progression. This will include ultrasound scanning, careful fluid balance and electrolyte monitoring.

Severe hyperstimulation is rare (less than 1% of cases) but serious. Breathing difficulties occur as fluid accumulates in the abdomen and chest. There is also a predisposition to thrombosis. This situation can be fatal and requires hospital admission and correction of fluid abnormalities.

Gonadotrophin hormone-releasing hormone analogue (GnRHa). GnRHa pumps secrete GnRH in a pulsatile manner, simulating the natural process. It may be administered subcutaneously or intravenously. The pump stimulates normal pituitary function, by substituting the hypothalamus and thereby stimulating normal follicular growth.

In theory there is no need to monitor follicular response, but hyperstimulation does occur and therefore the need to monitor as with gonadotrophin therapy is necessary.

Pregnancy rates in hypothalamic hypopituitary syndrome are good but no better than with HMG. GnRH pumps are better physiologically but there are no data to confirm that pregnancy rates are superior.

GnRH has been applied successfully for cases of hypogonadotrophic hypogonadism (e.g. Kallmann's syndrome), multicystic and polycystic ovaries.

GnRH analogue is equivalent to superphysiological doses and can be given either intranasally, subcutaneously or by implant. This allows down-regulation of the hypothalamic pituitary gonadal axis and reduction of endogenous gonadotrophin levels, and thus allows a 'sterile environment' for ovarian stimulation by HMG.

This treatment can be useful for patients with PCOS, recurrent aborters and is used on a routine basis in many assisted conception cycles.

Bromocriptine–dopamine agonists. Anovulation due to hyperprolactinaemia is associated with very favourable results after treatment. Ninety per cent will get pregnant within 3 months. Bromocriptine, a dopamine agonist, reduces the levels of prolactin and reduces the size and growth of prolactin-secreting adenomas. It is considered the treatment of choice, with recourse to surgery being rarely necessary. (Further details can be found in Chapter 4.)

Bromocriptine is usually started in doses of 2.5 mg b.d. and continued in a maintenance dose of 1.25 mg b.d. In cases of borderline levels of prolactin, bromocriptine has no role to play.

Treatment of uterine abnormalities

Disease of endometrium will prevent implantation and establishment of a pregnancy, and the commonest causes are endometrial atrophy, e.g. as a result of pelvic tuberculosis and Asherman's syndrome (intrauterine synechiae).

The diagnosis may be suggested by a hysterosalpingogram but is best made by hysteroscopy, with amenorrhoea being a presenting feature.

The hysteroscope has an important role in the investigation of the infertile woman. For patients with Mullerian tube abnormalities the role of metroplasty is debatable. Instances of infertility after metroplasty is in the region of 20–30% due to the associated development of Asherman's syndrome.

Cervical stenosis may cause infertility from a lack of mucus but dilatation has a very limited role in the treatment. Fibroids can cause infertility if they occlude the tubes. They can also be a cause of recurrent abortion. Myomectomies may have a role in treatment but are associated with very high rates of tubal disease due to infection, either clinical or subclinical.

Treatment of tubal disease

The incidence of tubal disease in an infertile population varies worldwide. In the UK it is estimated at 15%, in Singapore 11.7%, while in Cameroon it is 88%. In the UK there are about 8500 new cases of tubal disease per year.

The common causes are gonorrhoea, tuberculosis, bacteroides, other bacteria, chlamydia, mycoplasma, post-pregnancy/puerperal sepsis, IUCD, post-surgical. The association of IUCD with infertility is good enough reason to make it a contraindication to use it in nulliparous patients.

About 78% of patients with tubal disease will have had previous abdominal surgery. In 16% of these, it is an appendicectomy. Other procedures are salpingectomy for ectopic pregnancy, curettage and evacuation of retained products of conception. Twenty per cent of patients undergoing wedge resection of the ovary will develop tubal problems. Ventrosuspension performed for retroversion, which is not associated with infertility, may itself cause tubal disease.

The adequate treatment for tubal disease starts with prevention. Primary pelvic inflammatory disease should be accurately diagnosed by laparoscopy and treated vigorously with antibiotics to prevent residual disease. Triple therapy is required to cover aerobes, anaerobes and chlamydia.

The place of tubal surgery has been re-evaluated, with many opting for IVF as a first option, this being possibly an overall more cost-effective approach besides reducing patient discomfort and anxiety. However, until IVF is more widely available, tubal surgery will continue to be practised, especially for reversal of sterilisation. The results of surgery will depend upon patient selection (Table 5).

Treatment of endometriosis

Endometriosis has been fully discussed in Chapter 3. Endometriosis is present in 10–15% of pre-menopausal women undergoing gynaecological surgery. The behaviour of endometriosis is highly variable. The diagnosis of endometriosis depends on direct inspection of the peritoneum, not on history and examination, and laparoscopy is therefore mandatory.

Using a weighted point system, the American Fertility Society has proposed a classification system which distinguishes a minimal, mild–moderate and severe stage of the disease.

The association between infertility and endometriosis is not straightforward except in cases where there is anatomical distortion of the pelvic organs.

The management of endometriosis may be either medical, by hormone therapy, or surgical. Hormone therapy aims at suppressing ovarian activity and therefore withdrawing the stimulus for the endometriotic tissue, i.e. a

Table 5 Overall results of tubal surgery

Surgery performed	Pregnancy rate over 1 year
Salpingolysis	25–50%
Salpingostomy	20–25%
Tubal reimplantation	15–40%
Tubal reanastomosis	30–70%
Cornual block	15–30%
Reversal of sterilisation	
Microscopic surgery	90%
Macroscopic surgery	70%

pseudo-pregnancy or pseudo-menopause. A pseudo-pregnancy state can be created by either oral contraceptive or progestagens, while a pseudo-menopause is induced by danazol, gestrinone or GnRHa.

Withdrawal of hormone therapy may, however, be associated with reactivation of the disease. Furthermore fertility is postponed while on treatment. Surgical treatment is therefore to be considered as more definitive but this must be meticulous and excision of all diseased tissue is necessary. For infertile patients laparoscopic surgery is better than laparotomy as it is less likely to cause post-operative pelvic adhesions and tubal occlusion than laparotomy.

Simple endometriotic spots visualised at laparoscopy may be easily and definitely treated by simple diathermy or better still by laser vaporisation.

Treatment of unexplained infertility

This condition is frustrating because of lack of any cause to be found and the lack of specific treatment; 10–15% of couples attending a clinic will be labelled as suffering from unexplained infertility.

Treatment options include the following:

- *Nothing*. Couples with unexplained infertility of less than 3 years' duration are mostly normal and have simply been unlucky so far. Most will conceive within 2 years. Advice, explanation and reassurance are all that is needed. There is no simple treatment of benefit and unless the woman is over the age of 35 or has been trying for over 3 years a wait-and-see approach is best.
- *Superovulation and intrauterine insemination (IUI)*. This allows a greater recruitment of oocytes (maximum of three) and preparation of the sperm by a swim-up preparation. The prepared sperm is then inseminated into the uterus. Pregnancy rates of 15–20% per cycle have been reported. If

after 3 years an unexplained infertile couple have not conceived then up to three cycles of superovulation and IUI should be considered. This procedure requires large numbers of healthy sperm and is ineffective in cases of sperm disorder. The degree of superovulation has to be carefully monitored to reduce the risk of multiple pregnancy.

- *IVF and related assisted conception.* After more than 3 years the chance of natural conception offers unrealistic hope. IVF and related assisted conception methods now offer a substantial chance of success, with success virtually as good as normal in each cycle of treatment.

Results of treatment

As a result of non-assisted conception treatment about 18% of infertile couples can be expected to conceive. It is important to discuss this with the couples; the outcome of treatment is demonstrated in Figure 1.

Half the couples presenting with 1-year infertility can expect to become pregnant spontaneously in the following year. Figure 2 demonstrates the cumulative conception rates resulting from individual treatments as appropriate in women with amenorrhoea, and Figure 3 demonstrates cumulative conception rates in unexplained infertility without treatment related to duration of infertility when investigated.

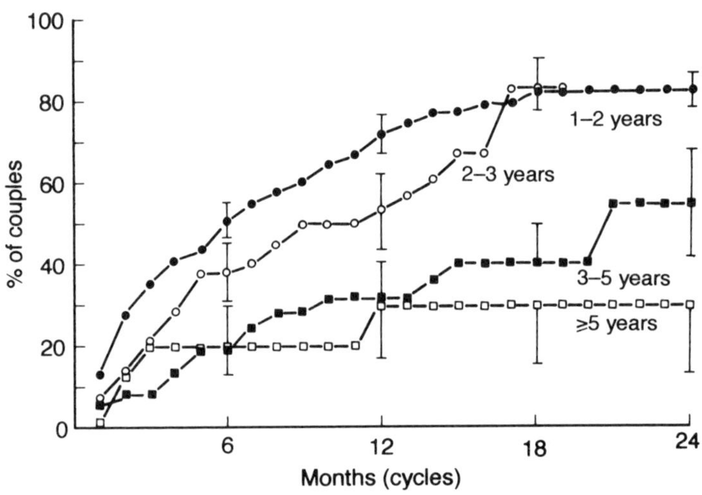

Figure 3 Cumulative conception rates in unexplained infertility without treatment related to duration of infertility when investigated. Reproduced from *British Medical Journal* 1985, **21**, 1693, with permission

Assisted conception

This is covered in depth in Chapter 6. The term 'assisted conception treatment' refers to methods that involve the stimulation of multiple ovulation and the delivery of specially prepared motile sperm to the eggs. The sperm and eggs may be mixed in the laboratory (IVF) or placed in the Fallopian tubes to fertilise—gamete intra-Fallopian transfer (GIFT).

Superovulation and intrauterine insemination are performed without surgical collection of eggs and prepared sperm is injected high into the uterus.

All assisted conception methods require normal fertilisation capacity and implantation.

With the birth of the first baby by IVF in 1978 the treatment of protracted infertility changed dramatically. The indications for assisted conception can be seen in Table 6.

In the UK success rates are monitored by the Human Fertilisation and Embryology Authority. Table 7 records the success rates for 1990 and Table 8 gives success rates by age for IVF.

Table 6 Indications for assisted conception as advised by the Fertility Committee of the Royal College of Obstetricians and Gynaecologists (1992)

Tubes	Sperm	Ovaries	Pathology	Treatment
Patent	Normal	Accessible Normal	Unexplained PCOS	IUI with super-ovulation GIFT IVF
Patent	Absent	Accessible Normal	Azoospermia Male genetic disease	DI Donor GIFT Donor IVF
Patent	Poor	Accessible	Oligozoo-spermia Terato/asthenozoo-spermia	IVF ZIFT[a] GIFT Micromanipu-lation
Absent/damaged	Normal/poor	Accessible Normal	Tubal disease Severe endometri-osis	IVF
Patent/absent	Normal	Non-functional Absent	Ovarian failure Oophor-ectomy Female genetic disease	Donor oocyte GIFT (patent tubes) Donor oocyte IVF

[a] ZIFT = zygote intra-Fallopian transfer.

Table 7 Success rates by indications for treatment 1990

Pathology	Pregnancy rates (%)		Live birth rates (%)	
	Per cycle	Per transfer	Per cycle	Per transfer
Tubal	18.3	24.1	12.7	16.8
Endometriosis	18.0	25.5	13.7	19.4
Male factor	15.9	24.6[a]	11.3	17.4[a]
Unexplained	15.3	22.2	11.8	17.1
Cervical factors	15.1	21.7	10.9	15.5
Ovarian and other	17.1	25	12.7	18.6

[a] Includes cases in which donor sperm used (HFEA, 1992).

Table 8 IVF success rate by woman's age 1990

	Under 25	25–29	30–34	35–39	40–44	45+
Pregnancy rate (%)						
Per cycle	15.9	20.9	19.6	16.2	7.8	2.9
Per transfer	24.2	27.3	26.2	23.0	12.3	4.9
Live birth rate (%)						
Per cycle	9.7	15.2	14.7	11.4	4.0	0.0
Per transfer	14.8	19.9	19.8	16.0	6.3	0.0

Reproductive technologies are discussed in depth in Chapter 6.

CONCLUSION

Infertility is a common problem affecting up to one in six couples who wish to conceive.

A proper work-up includes a full history, examination and appropriate investigations.

Stress is an important problem and needs to be overcome as far as possible.

Early referral to specialist centres is important to allow the couple to take advantage of some of the assisted conception techniques now available.

SUGGESTED READING

Abdalla, H., Baber, R. and Studd, J. (1990). The active management of infertility. In J. Studd (ed.), *Progress in Obstetrics and Gynaecology*, Vol. 8, Churchill Livingstone, Edinburgh, pp. 273–287.

American Fertility Society (1985). Revised classification of endometriosis. *Fertil. Steril.*, **43**, 351.

Hewitt, J., Cohen, J. and Steptoe, P. (1987). Male infertility and in vitro fertilisation. In J. Studd (ed.), *Progress in Obstetrics and Gynaecology*, Vol. 6, Churchill Livingstone, Edinburgh, pp. 253–275.

Hull, M. R., Glazener, C. M. A., Kelley, N. J., Conway, D. I., Foster, P. A., Hinton, R. A., Coulsan, C., Lambert, P. A. and Watt, E. M. (1985). Population studies of causes, treatment and outcome of infertility. *Br. Med. J.*, **291**, 1693–1697.

Human Fertilisation and Embryology Authority Annual Report (1992). HFEA.

Infertility Guidelines for Practice (1992). RCOG Press.

Lilford, R. J. and Watson, A. J. (1990). Has IVF made salpingostomy obsolete? *Obstet. Gynaecol.*, **97**, 557–560.

Mishell, R. D., Davajan, Y. and Lobo, R. (1991). *Infertility, Contraception and Reproductive Endocrinology*, 3rd edn. Blackwell Scientific Publications, Oxford.

Winston, R. (1981). Tubal microsurgery. In J. Studd (ed.), *Progress in Obstetrics and Gynaecology*. pp. 291–303.

6

Assisted Reproductive Technologies

Jane L. Frederick and Ricardo H. Asch
University of California, Irvine, California, USA

In Chapter 5 an introduction to assisted reproductive technologies (ART) was given. In this chapter a more detailed account of the different techniques is provided.

GAMETE INTRA-FALLOPIAN TRANSFER

Gamete intra-Fallopian transfer (GIFT) is a technique devised to achieve pregnancies in couples who have not been able to conceive using conventional treatments for infertility (Asch et al., 1986). Essentially the name explains the procedure. Gametes—the female's egg and male's sperm—are placed separately into a catheter and injected directly into the woman's Fallopian tubes during a surgical procedure. Fertilisation occurs in the woman's body, not outside or *in vitro* in a laboratory dish or in an incubator. GIFT mimics the way a normally fertilised egg would begin its journey to the uterus for implantation. The GIFT procedure follows nature by allowing the eggs to fertilise and develop in the natural environment of the Fallopian tube, and then to make their way to the uterus for implantation according to a normal timetable.

To prepare her body for the GIFT procedure, the woman receives hormones to stimulate development of the ovarian follicles, which are sac-like structures that contain the unfertilised eggs (Table 1). Administering hormones increases the chances of retrieving several ripened eggs, each capable of being fertilised by sperm once transferred to the tubes. Most commonly in our institution we utilise a combination of gonadotrophin-releasing

Understanding Common Disorders in Reproductive Endocrinology. Edited by M.M. Dooley and M.P. Brincat.

Table 1 Chronology of a GIFT cycle

1. Induction of follicular development
2. HCG administration
3. Sperm preparation
4. Oocyte pick-up
5. Oocyte identification
6. Gamete loading and transfer
7. Luteal phase support
8. Diagnosis of pregnancy

hormone agonist (GnRHa) beginning in the luteal phase and pure follicle-stimulating hormone (FSH) and human menopausal gonadotrophins (HMG), or a combination of clomiphene citrate (CC) and HMG. Follicular maturation is assessed by periodic vaginal ultrasounds and serum oestradiol levels (E_2). Human chorionic gonadotrophin (HCG) 10 000 IU is given when a minimum of two or three follicles have a maximum diameter of at least 20 mm when utilising the GnRHa/FSH/HMG protocol, and when a leading follicle has a largest diameter of 18 mm with the CC/HMG protocol. Oocyte retrieval is carried out 34–36 h after HCG injection.

Approximately 2 h before the procedure, a semen sample is obtained from the husband. In the laboratory, the semen sample is prepared by a technique of 'wash and swim up'. This means the semen is centrifuged, washed with a culture medium and placed in a test tube. Most of the sperm settle on the bottom, but the most active ones, those that 'swim' to the top, are selected and loaded into the catheter.

The eggs can be retrieved from the follicles in the ovary in several ways: some of them surgical (laparoscopy, culdoscopy, mini-laparotomy) and some non-surgical (ultrasound-guided aspiration).

After aspiration of the follicles, the fluids are examined under a microscope by a trained biologist and their maturity determined. Eggs and sperm are then sequentially and separately loaded into a catheter and are then placed into each of the patient's Fallopian tubes. This can be achieved by several methods, the more common being laparoscopy or mini-laparotomy.

When the catheter is in place in the Fallopian tube, the eggs and sperm are injected into the tube using a special syringe. The catheter is loaded with two to four oocytes and 100 000+ sperm in a total volume of 50 μl or less. If both tubes appear normal, transfer is carried out to each tube. If one tube is difficult to cannulate, transfer is made to the 'good' tube only. Generally three to five oocytes in total are transferred, depending on the patient's age, oocyte maturity, etc. In the UK, owing to the Human Fertilisation and Embryology Authority (HFEA) guidelines, three or in very exceptional circumstances four oocytes can be replaced. If possible, gametes are transferred at least 3–4 cm into the fimbriated end of the tube. The transferred gametes come together in the Fallopian tubes, where the fertilisation process is allowed to happen naturally. The resulting embryos are nurtured in the tubes, then move down into the uterus for implantation (Figure 1).

The GIFT technique is performed as a one-step procedure. The entire procedure lasts approximately 40–60 min, and the patient returns home the same day. Pregnancy can be confirmed using blood and urine tests approximately 10–12 days after GIFT, and by ultrasound approximately 25 days after GIFT. The luteal phase is supported with 50 mg of progesterone intramuscularly daily, and if pregnancy occurs progesterone is continued until 6 weeks from transfer.

One of the originally described pre-requisites for a GIFT cycle has been at least one patent Fallopian tube. Most clinicians will not perform GIFT in a patent tube that appears abnormal. Similarly most clinicians feel that previous surgery on a Fallopian tube, such as for an ectopic pregnancy or neosalpingostomy and even tubal reanastomosis, is a contraindication to GIFT. The fear in these cases is that either the tube will not function normally for gamete transport and the procedure will be unsuccessful or ectopic pregnancy will result.

TUBAL EMBRYO TRANSFER

GIFT was originally developed as a therapeutic alternative for patients with at least one functional Fallopian tube. In most investigators' experience its efficacy has proven superior to *in vitro* fertilisation (IVF) in couples with most categories of infertility. Unfortunately, success rates with GIFT in cases of significant male factor infertility are lower than with other aetiologies. In these cases, IVF offers the advantage of exposing the oocytes to high concentrations of motile sperm and, in addition, diagnostically, offers the definitive answer to the question of fertilisation. The implantation rate in GIFT is, however, superior to that in IVF, theoretically because of the effect of the intratubal milieu on early development and the more chronologically appropriate entrance of the embryo into the uterus. The concept of tubal embryo transfer (TET) was therefore explored as a hybrid of both GIFT and IVF.

Devroey et al. reported on the first successful case of tubal embryo transfer in a patient with antisperm antibodies in 1986. He termed the transfer a zygote intra-Fallopian transfer (ZIFT). Transfer was performed 18 h after insemination, hence the designation zygote. In 1987 Yovich et al. reported their results in a series of patients undergoing pronuclear stage tubal transfer (PROST). This technique was utilised in cases of severe male factor, female antisperm antibodies, poor results from multiple previous GIFT cycles, and in women receiving donated oocytes. Results were superior to

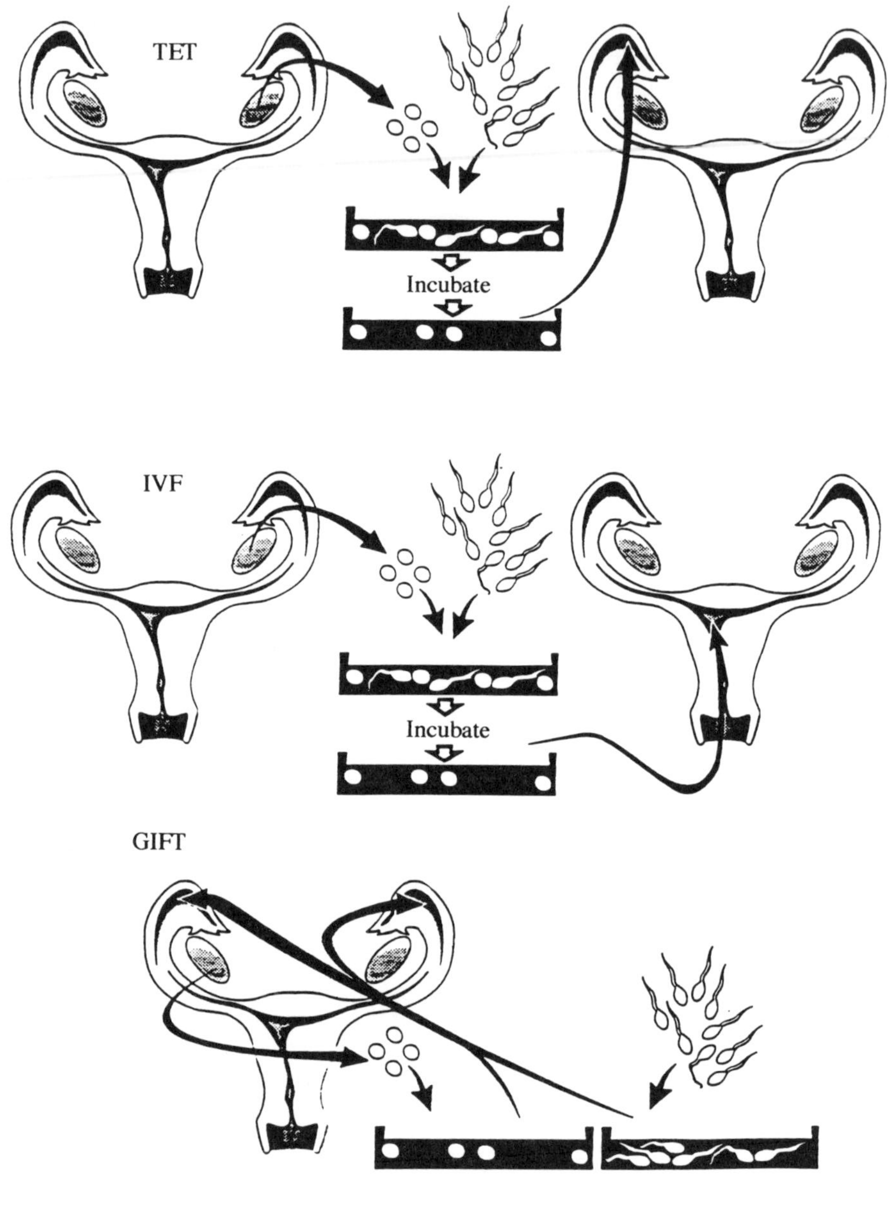

Figure 1

IVF. The authors commented that the diagnostic value of PROST was clearly demonstrated by the confirmation of fertilisation failure in many severe male factor couples. These couples can then be counselled as to future therapy. Yovich et al. concluded that PROST is a superior technique as compared with IVF for managing cases of severe male factor and female antisperm antibodies. In their discussion they comment that in couples who have failed multiple previous GIFT cycles, use of PROST which documents fertilisation only may be inferior to TET which contributes additional knowledge regarding cleavage and early embryo development.

In 1988 Balmaceda et al. reported our preliminary results with TET in cases of male factor. Sixteen couples began a TET cycle. Following controlled ovarian hyperstimulation and transvaginal oocyte retrieval, insemination was performed. No fertilisation occurred in six cases. In the remaining 10 patients, TET was performed 45–50 hours after oocyte retrieval. This time interval was chosen based on information obtained in an experimental model in non-human primates. Six pregnancies occurred, including one twin and one triplet. The implantation rate of 25.7% was superior to the 7–10% implantation rate expected from uterine transfer. In an article comparing the relative chance of pregnancy following tubal or uterine transfer procedures, Yovich et al. (1988a) similarly reported that the pregnancy rate per transfer and the implantation rates were significantly higher for tubal transfer. Devroey et al. in 1989 presented their data on 245 ZIFT cycles. They had a 43% pregnancy rate from transferring three or less zygotes.

Results of TET at our centre to date have shown 67 pregnancies in 126 transfers, for a 53% pregnancy rate per transfer. Of interest is the implantation rate of 18% per embryo transferred as compared with the 7–10% rate quoted for uterine transfer. Miscarriage and multiple birth rates are similar to those reported with IVF and GIFT. Thus it appears that TET is quite promising in male factor and immunological infertility when compared with GIFT (16%) and IVF (12%).

Although the pregnancy rate per transfer in our centre is 53%, many severe male factor patients do not make it to transfer because of a failure of fertilisation (pregnancy rate of 28% · per cycle attempted). Methods are needed to improve sperm recovery and fertilisation in severe male factor cases. Yovich et al. (1988b) reported on the use of the phosphodiesterase inhibitor pentoxifylline (PF) to enhance the number of progressively motile sperm available for insemination. An *in vitro* trial demonstrated an improvement in concentration of motile spermatozoa and progressively motile sperm in oligospermic samples for PF treatment. PF washing of sperm was then carried out in nine couples who had previously failed attempts at fertilisation *in vitro*. Six couples achieved fertilisation with PF-treated sperm and five pregnancies ensued following PROST. Further study of this promising treatment is needed.

In our centre, we have obtained good sperm recovery in cases of severe male factor using the mini-percoll technique. Semen samples are collected and diluted 1:2 with medium and then centrifuged at 200 × *g* for 10 min. Pellets are suspended in 0.3 ml of medium (human tubal fluid (HTF) and Hepes, Irvine Scientific, California) and layered on a discontinuous percoll (Pharmacia, Sweden) gradient consisting of 0.3 ml each of 50%, 70% and 95% isotonic percoll (mini-percoll). The gradient is centrifuged at 300 × *g* for 45 min. Following centrifugation the 95% percoll layer is removed, washed two times and resuspended in 1 ml of HTF and 10% human cord serum. Cumulus denuded oocytes are then added to the culture tube containing sperm. In our comparative study with a standard swim-up technique, semen samples prepared with the mini-percoll technique had a better motility and progression, and normal morphology. In addition the fertilisation rate and pregnancy rate were superior in the mini-percoll group. Based on our preliminary data, the mini-percoll technique for sperm preparation seems to offer significant advantages in cases of severe oligoasthenospermia.

Our present policy for triaging patients for assisted reproductive technology (ART) cycles includes utilising TET for four indications: (1) severe male factor; (2) immunological infertility; (3) previous failed GIFT cycle; and (4) immature eggs obtained at the time of a GIFT cycle.

Prior to beginning an ART cycle a semen analysis with preparation of the sample is obtained. If the following criteria are not met TET rather than GIFT becomes our method of choice:

1. Recovery of >1.5 million total motile sperm.
2. Sperm progression in the forward direction.
3. Percentage of normal forms >30%.

Any sperm preparation not fulfilling these criteria is considered a male factor, and TET is recommended.

In cases of female antisperm antibodies, TET rather than GIFT is performed. In these couples female sera are not used for culture, and fertilisation takes place outside the body.

Any couple who have previously undergone a GIFT cycle in our programme and fail to achieve a pregnancy are also triaged to TET in the following cycle. In this way we (1) find out about fertilisation, and (2) put back only fertilised eggs rather than some that may not fertilise (may occur in a GIFT cycle). Even when supernumerary oocytes have fertilised in a previous GIFT cycle, we prefer to do a TET cycle.

Finally, in cases scheduled for GIFT in which we obtain fewer than three mature oocytes, the GIFT is cancelled and insemination is delayed and performed *in vitro*. If two or more embryos are obtained TET is then carried out. This policy is based on data demonstrating that the pregnancy rate is significantly poorer when immature eggs are transferred for GIFT. The tube seems to be a good place for embryo development, but not for oocyte maturation.

We feel that by utilising this policy of patient selection for GIFT versus TET we are able to diagnose a failure of fertilisation in many cases of severe male factor and thus not subject the woman to surgery (GIFT) unless embryos are obtained. Furthermore, as micromanipulation techniques improve, TET will be the transfer method of choice in these couples when the woman has functional tubes.

OOCYTE DONATION AND TUBAL TRANSFER

The first successful case of oocyte donation in ART was reported by Lutjen et al. in 1984. IVF and embryo transfer of donated oocytes was performed on a woman with premature ovarian failure (POF). Presently indications for donated oocytes include POF, carriers of a lethal genetic trait, as well as women with a history of a reported poor response in previous ART cycles. Since Lutjen's original report many investigators have described oocyte donation for IVF cycles, with uniformly good success rates of 25–35%. In 1988 Asch et al. reported the first series of oocyte donation in GIFT cycles, with six of eight patients conceiving. Subsequently, Formigli et al. (1989) reported similarly excellent results from oocyte donation in GIFT cycles. Yovich et al. suggested the use of PROST for oocyte donation cycles. They recommended PROST because: (1) in general results of tubal transfer were superior to uterine transfer in their programme; and (2) transfer of pronuclear stage embryos allowed for a separation in time between oocyte aspiration and transfer that preserved anonymity of donors (more difficult with GIFT). Success was similarly good.

Presently our protocol for oocyte recipients includes an evaluation cycle in which they receive the following steroid replacement: (1) micronised 17β-oestradiol (E_2) orally (Estrace, Mead Johnson, Evansville, Indiana) 2 mg on days 3–8, 4 mg on days 9–11, and 6 mg on days 12–28, in divided daily doses; and (2) progesterone (P) in oil intramuscularly IM (United Research Laboratories, Philadelphia, Pennsylvania) 100 mg/day, days 16–28. Serum E_2 and P levels are determined by radioimmunoassay on days 8, 11, 15 and 20 of the evaluation cycle and an endometrial biopsy is performed in the mid- to late luteal phase. During the cycle of oocyte donation all recipients follow a similar steroid replacement regimen based on results from the evaluation cycle. P is begun 2 days prior to gamete or embryo transfer. If pregnancy results, E_2 8 mg and P 100 mg daily is continued until 60 days from transfer.

In a recent report from our centre, Rotszetjn et al. (1990) presented data comparing pregnancy rates with oocyte donation in cases of IVF, GIFT and TET. Our present results suggest that in cases of oocyte donation there is no significant difference in outcome between IVF and ZIFT. However, although the number of cases of GIFT is small, the pregnancy rate and implantation rate appear to be slightly higher than that with IVF. We are presently carrying out a prospective randomised study of IVF versus GIFT for oocyte donation. If in fact GIFT proves superior, then all patients with a functional Fallopian tube should be offered GIFT for oocyte donation. The patient will then need to decide whether the increased chance of pregnancy with GIFT compensates for the necessity of a surgical procedure (mini-laparotomy or laparoscopy) as opposed to non-surgical transfer with IVF.

GAMETE INTRA-FALLOPIAN TRANSFER IN COMBINATION WITH *IN VITRO* FERTILISATION

GIFT is now an established technique for assisted conception in couples where the woman has a patent Fallopian tube. IVF, although having a lower success rate, does provide more immediate answers with regard to fertilisation capacity. Therefore it was natural that some investigators would propose a combined procedure of GIFT and IVF to provide more information and give a higher chance of pregnancy. In the combined approach GIFT is carried out in a routine fashion, and 2–3 days later embryos obtained from fertilisation of excess oocytes are transferred to the uterus.

Leong et al. (1988) reported on a small study comparing GIFT with a combined GIFT/IVF approach. They found a lower pregnancy rate with the combined approach (10% versus 39%). They conclude that GIFT and IVF are neither compatible nor complementary. Theories as to why pregnancy rates are lower with the combined approach include: (1) the uterine embryo transfer may cause trauma to the endometrium, preventing implantation of embryos travelling down the Fallopian tubes originating from GIFT; (2) if uterine transferred embryos do not survive, toxins may be released that might kill the embryos still in the tube; or (3) the uterine transferred embryos may initiate implantation (even if they do not ultimately result in a pregnancy) and this may prevent further development and implantation of Fallopian tube embryos.

The 1988 IVF–ET Registry for the United States reported an overall 27% clinical pregnancy rate for GIFT and an overall 25% clinical pregnancy rate for combined GIFT/IVF. With the increasing availability of cryopreservation, it seems as though supernumerary embryos obtained from a GIFT cycle should be cryopreserved for future use rather than transferred to the uterus during the GIFT cycle. Preliminary data would suggest that even in programmes where cyropreservation is not an option, transferring excess embryos to the uterus in a GIFT cycle may be detrimental.

IN VITRO FERTILISATION

IVF was first developed as a method of treating tubal infertility in women with absent Fallopian tubes or uncorrectable tubal disease. However, with time, the indications have been extended to any infertility aetiology not amenable to conventional therapy. Thus, IVF is commonly utilised to treat the following specific indications: tubal disease (the most common), endometriosis, male infertility, unexplained infertility, diethylstilboestrol (DES) exposure, cervical factor and immunological infertility.

Increasing experience with IVF has suggested that the expected pregnancy rate is similar regardless of the infertility diagnosis; further, the pregnancy rate is not diminished in patients with multiple aetiologies. Although these facts are generally true, we have now identified specific subgroups of patients with a variety of clinical diagnoses in whom there is an impairment in reproductive potential; this is especially relevant among the male factor population with severe teratozoospermia.

The overall IVF pregnancy rate of 25–30% per embryo transfer (for all factors of infertility) is remarkably similar to the pregnancy rate following 1 month of exposure during normal reproduction. Thus, it can be concluded that IVF and embryo transfer can now be accepted as a standard and successful clinical therapy for a variety of conditions.

Tubal infertility continues to be the major indications for IVF. Success of treatment is not related to severity of tubo-ovarian disease. Early experience with laparoscopic retrievals suggested that patients with severe tubo-ovarian disease (with inaccessible ovaries) had a somewhat poorer outcome than patients with milder disease. With the use of ultrasonographic aspiration, almost all ovaries are accessible to aspiration. Thus, there are no differences in the number of pre-ovulatory oocytes, fertilisation rates or ongoing pregnancy rates relative to severity of disease. However, patients who have had prior tubal ligations (with no organic disease and previously proven fertility) exhibit higher peak oestradiol responses to stimulation and higher pregnancy rates than patients with failed tuboplasty or bilateral salpingectomies.

The IVF cycle is conducted in an identical manner to the GIFT/ZIFT cycles. In particular, regimens of controlled ovarian hyperstimulation are identical, as is the method of oocyte retrieval, fertilisation and embryo culture. The only difference is the method of embryo transfer in IVF, in which a small catheter is used to transfer the embryos transcervically to the uterus. In this instance, no anaesthesia or surgical intervention is necessary.

SUGGESTED READING

Asch, R. H., Bałmaceda, J. P., Ellsworth, L. R. and Wong, P. C. (1986). Preliminary experiences with GIFT (gamete intra fallopian transfer). *Fertil. Steril.*, **45**, 366.

Asch, R. H., Balmaceda, J. P., Ord, T. et al. (1988). Oocyte donation and gamete intrafallopian transfer in premature ovarian failure. *Fertil. Steril.*, **49**, 263–267.

Balmaceda, J. P., Gastaldi, C., Remohi, J., Borrero, C., Ord, T. and Asch, R. H. (1988). Tubal embryo transfer as a treatment for infertility due to male factor. *Fertil. Steril.*, **50**, 476–479.

Devroey, P., Braeckmans, P., Smith, J. et al. (1986). Pregnancy after translaparoscopic zygote intrafallopian transfer in a patient with sperm antibodies. *Lancet*, **i**, 1329.

Devroey, P., Camus, M., Stuessen, C. et al. (1989). ZIFT: indications and limitations. In Capitano, G. L., Asch, R. H., DeCecco, L. and Croce, S. (eds), *GIFT: From Basics to Clinics.* Raven Press, New York.

Formigli, L., Roccio, C., Belotti, G., Stangalini, A., Coglitore, M. T. and Formigli, G. (1989). Oocyte donation by gamete intrafallopian transfer to amenorrheic and cycling patients given replacement steroids. *Human Reprod.*, **4**, 772–776.

Leong, M. K. H., Leung, C. K. M., Marriott, V. M. *et al.* (1988). Comparative study of combined GIFT and IVF–ET with GIFT alone. *Human Reprod.*, **9**, 877–879.

Lutjen, P., Trounson, A., Leeton, J., Findlay, J., Wood, C. and Renou, P. (1984). The establishment and maintenance of pregnancy using in vitro fertilization and embryo donation in a patient with primary ovarian failure. *Nature*, **307**, 174–175.

Medical Research International and the Society for Assisted Reproductive Technology, The American Fertility Society (1991). In vitro fertilization—embryo transfer in the United States: 1989 results from the IVF–ET Registry. *Fertil. Steril.*, **55**, 14–23.

Rotszetjn, D. A., Remohi, J., Borrero, C., Ord, T., Balmaceda, J. P. and Asch, R. H. (1990). Oocyte donation with GIFT, IVF–UT or TET: is there a best alternative? Presented at the Forty-Sixth Annual Meeting of the American Fertility Society, October 13–18, 1990, Washington, DC.

Yovich, J. L., Blackledge, D. G., Richardson, P. A., Matson, P. L., Turner, S. R. and Draper, R. (1987). Pregnancies following pronuclear stage tubal transfer. *Fertil. Steril.*, **48**, 851–857.

Yovich, J. L., Yovich, J. M. and Edirisinghe, W. R. (1988a) The relative chance of pregnancy following tubal or uterine transfer procedures. *Fertil. Steril.*, **49**, 858–864.

Yovich, J. M., Edirisinghe, W. R., Cummins, J. M. and Yovich, J. L. (1988b). Preliminary results using pentoxifylline in a pronuclear stage tubal transfer (PROST) program for severe male factor infertility. *Fertil. Steril.*, **50**, 179–181.

7

Moral Issues in Assisted Conception

Neil Pickering
Centre for the Study of Philosophy and Health Care, University College, Swansea, UK

The question which this chapter will address is whether there may be moral justifications for refusing to provide assisted conception.

To address this issue, it will be necessary to go beyond questions of what should or should not be done when treating infertility (ethical or moral questions). For instance, a confusion about ethics in infertility treatment may arise from a confusion about what infertility actually is, about the definition of the word, and about whether or not it is the appropriate word to use in talking about the moral issues within reproductive medicine. Reflection on the meaning or definition of words may be termed philosophical or conceptual reflection—although there is no guarantee that ethical uncertainty will be clarified by such 'conceptual' reflection.

Throughout this chapter there will be reference to cases of the kind which may give rise to moral concern in assisted reproduction, causing health carers to wonder 'Is it appropriate to treat this person?' Each of these examples is modelled upon an actual case.

The chapter has three main sections. The first analyses moral doubts and concerns such as whether it is right to help all people who request help to conceive. The second and third sections ask if moral justifications may be found for translating such doubts in the mind into practice, and for refusing to treat some clients.

It is important to make clear that these will be possible justifications, and that whether they are morally persuasive will depend on the weight which they carry, and that in turn will rest upon people's experiences and deeply held beliefs.

Understanding Common Disorders in Reproductive Endocrinology. Edited by M.M. Dooley and M.P. Brincat.

MORAL QUESTIONS THAT MAY ARISE IN PRACTICE

This section is concerned with the kinds of moral doubts that may trouble health carers, and that may make them doubt the appropriateness of helping a certain patient. What might be the nature of such doubts? What might they rest on?

Suppose Mrs S requests infertility treatment. She is over 50 years old, yet still ovulating. She has come (or been referred) to the infertility services as her only option for conceiving. She is too old to be accepted for adoption; a widow, without a partner.

A question may arise as to whether it is right to help Mrs S. It may arise even if the clinic believes she is unlikely to be able to have a child. For even if tests showed her to be unlikely successfully to carry to term a baby, an argument can be made out for treating her on the grounds that it may relieve her distress to do so. In other words, while clinical facts may suggest it is impossible to treat the primary feature of someone's infertility (childlessness), it may be possible to treat or alleviate other symptoms such as unhappiness. The moral issues that might trouble a health carer in such a case would be different from those which are the main focus of this chapter, which are those that may arise where having a child is possible and is intended.

Some other kinds of facts (other than clinical facts, that is) may lie behind doubts as to whether or not it is appropriate to try and help Mrs S have a baby. She is over 50, and women can expect to live in excess of 70 years; but her risk of dying before any child born now matures is much greater than with a younger mother. If she were to die that would be traumatic for the child, and leaving it without a parent might badly affect its upbringing. She will also get less fit as she ages, which might be especially difficult if she is on her own. Moreover, the risk of conceiving a handicapped child is higher for a woman in her fifties than for a woman of a younger age group. These facts may seem to lead directly to doubts about what might be the appropriate response to Mrs S. But would such doubts be based entirely on these facts?

They would not. In general terms, this is because the doubts mentioned must involve ideas about the meaning of certain words (conceptual ideas) and, in addition, must involve moral values connected with those ideas. This point is easier seen initially in the context of a second case.

Ms J is 25, presents as infertile, without a partner but in an unsteady relationship. Suppose a health carer considers that this is an unstable home life for a baby, and that it is wrong to offer assisted conception.

While the facts about Ms J's life may seem to be the basis of this moral judgement, it is not obvious that they constitute a picture of instability. This depends on what 'instability' and 'stability' are thought to mean; does stability require one partner only, living in, and preferably married to Ms J? Also assumed is the idea that it is wrong to bring up a child in an unstable home. That in turn may imply the belief (or value) that children should at least be given an adequate upbringing, and therefore a stable home background is necessary.

This general moral sentiment, that children deserve to have an adequate upbringing, may also underlie doubts as to whether or not to help Mrs S. In her case, doubts about treatment are based in part upon the statistical risk of her early death before the child is independent. A health carer who thinks in these terms must also hold that for a child to have an adequate upbringing it must have a genetic mother (or perhaps, one parent) to care for her until a certain maturity or age.

In addition, it is feared that, because of her age, Mrs S may have a handicapped child. Such a child could be so badly disadvantaged if born that it may be thought impossible for it to have an acceptable sort of life. Such a view would rest upon some idea of what an 'acceptable' sort of life might be (which is a conceptual matter); and upon the belief that it is right to help create only lives of sufficiently acceptable quality (a moral belief).

These, then, are the kinds of issue which may give rise to a feeling that certain clients should be refused help to have a child. What seems to lie behind the question of whether or not it is appropriate to help either Mrs S or Ms J is a concern for the child. The health carer who feels such doubts seems to be taking into account the interests not only of her patient (Mrs S, for instance) but also of the child Mrs S may have. These become doubts about treating Mrs S when the interests of the child and the interests of Mrs S cannot both be realised.

Should health carer teams or individuals act upon these doubts, and refuse treatment? Is there justification for acting upon these concerns in that way?

THE INTERESTS OF THE CHILD

The principal objection to acting upon such doubts by refusing treatment to some few clients is that it is wrong to do so. Such an objection claims that good practice in assisted reproduction entails putting aside concerns for the interests of the child where they clash with the interests of the client, and always helping the client. Against that is the argument that concern for the possible child is always appropriate, should be expressed, and may form the basis of a refusal to help.

The principal justification for the latter argument is that the work of those in assisted reproduction is peculiar in a particular and significant way. It is sometimes called assisted conception, but assisted reproduction is more accurate in those contexts which are of primary concern here. Where the aim of such treatment is the birth of a baby, that baby's well-being is of moral concern. Thus, this argument goes, the health carer who is (necessarily) involved in the conception of this child has some degree of responsibility to the child. The patient should not be the health carer's only concern. (Indeed, it is a somewhat moot point exactly who the patient is!)

This is recognised legislatively in the UK in the Human Fertilisation and Embryology Act (1990), which also makes it clear that the assessment of the child's interests must be multidisciplinary (that is, considerations other than the clinical should be taken into account where relevant).

The argument for taking into account the interests of the child in assisted reproduction asserts further that these interests may be of overriding moral concern. In other words, such interests may compel a health carer not to treat Mrs S, even though there are other moral arguments showing she should be treated, for instance that she is desperately unhappy without a child.

In which situations is a potential child's interest contrary to that of its potential parent? The refusal to intervene so as to help a woman bear a child is necessarily a refusal to bring about a life. Generally speaking, it seems that bringing about a life would be a good thing to do.

What would make it a bad thing to do? Or, to put it another way, what kind of consideration could form a justification for not bringing about a life? The principal point to be made here is that different considerations may properly arise at this point (before conception) from those which may justifiably arise after conception. That there may be some difference in our attitudes in the two situations can be illustrated by an example.

Suppose, after being helped to conceive, Ms J came into hospital with complications of her pregnancy, and in danger of losing the baby. Would there be any hesitation to help her on grounds such as those earlier mentioned, for instance that the baby might live an unstable home life? In fact, it is highly unlikely that such information would be sought, let alone acted upon.

Does this show that questions to elicit this information were (necessarily) inappropriate when Ms J came for help to conceive? It does not, for the situation is fundamentally different in the case of the complication of pregnancy—a life already exists. That difference may morally be decisive, in the sense that certain interests of the unborn (a stable home) which seem no justification for failing to save its life (a far more weighty interest) might be justification for not helping there to be a life in the first place.

Thus far, the idea that there could be any justifications for any such action and that they could override the interests of Mrs S is simply an assertion that will need to be tested. I consider three objections: first, that it is always wrong for health carers to make moral judgements about the choices of clients in assisted reproduction; second, that there is an overriding moral justification for helping people who present with supposed infertility; and third, that infertility is a disease which, like any other disease, it is a duty of the health carer to treat if she can.

The nub of each objection is that the health carer is primarily responsible to the clients, so that the interests of the child (whatever they might be) cannot be morally overriding. It follows from this that the assertion—that concern for a child may form the basis of a refusal to treat—made earlier is false. Surviving these objections will not show this assertion is correct, but will give grounds for considering it to have some strength. In that case, it may be a justification for actually refusing to treat Mrs S, Ms J, or others in some circumstances. (It is important to stress again that the weight moral arguments have for individuals and for societies rests mainly upon the depth to which people feel them or their foundations to be true.)

One moral judgement cannot be better than another

The first objection might be put like this: Mrs S has made a choice to have a child, and she has come to the infertility unit in order to do so. Moral objections to her as a mother may come to mind, but they cannot form a justification for overriding her choice, and refusing to help her. This is because she herself is making a moral judgement in choosing this course of action, and one moral judgement cannot override another.

One strength of this objection is that it reflects a view that is quite widely held. Mary Midgely discusses it in *Can't We Make Moral Judgements?*, although she argues against it. Put colloquially, the view is sometimes expressed thus: people who make moral judgements about others are nosey, do-gooders, and patronising—which is, as Midgely points out, a moral judgement itself. At heart this view, more accurately expressed, is that no one person's moral judgement is better than another.

The view that all moral judgements are of equal worth may rest upon any one of several other assumptions about what moral judgements actually are (what the words 'moral judgement' mean). One such assumption is that all moral judgements are, in the end, personal and private, arising out of gut reactions, intuitions, and so forth. On this account, the contradictory moral views of Mrs S and a health carer who may think it wrong to help her conceive are neither more justifiable than the other. Each person happens to have her own moral opinion, they happen to be contradictory, and there is not much more to be said on the matter.

If this view is correct, then it follows that there can be no moral justification for setting up institutions that give power to one moral opinion over another. Hence, it is wrong that the infertility unit should give to the doctors and nurses a power to refuse assisted reproduction to any client. (By the same token, of course, there is no reason why Mrs S's desire should be met.)

But is this account (or description) of moral judgements correct? In fact, even if it could be shown that they were merely personal, and not very rational to boot, it would not follow that it was wrong to choose whom to treat. This is because moral beliefs, however they originate, must involve the possibility of making serious negative judgements about others.

For example, suppose a health carer believes that it is wrong to bring into the world a child for which there will be no proper provision of care or love. What account can be given of her meaning? It cannot be that the health carer thinks it wrong to do so, but nonetheless also thinks that others who differ in their views are just as right as she. If she thought like that, then it would not be correct to describe hers as a moral view at all. Instead, it is more like a trivial opinion, on a par with a guess about which horse will win a race. (The health carer might well admit that 'your guess is as good as mine'.)

This does not show that it would be right for the health carer to act in accordance with her belief, and deny Mrs S, or anyone else, help to have a child. The belief might itself be controversial. It does suggest that those who hold moral beliefs will feel they should act in accordance with them. Thus, although the judgement may in some sense be a personal one, the health carer who holds that it is wrong to help Mrs S will tend to feel it is important to act in accordance with her judgement.

Moral beliefs, by their very nature, involve judgements about other people, and the possibility of acting in accordance with those judgements. In some cases, the justifications may be so strong in the mind of a health carer as to be overriding, compelling her to refuse help.

All clients for assisted reproduction must be helped

The second objection is this: a powerful moral reason for treating Mrs S and all other clients for assisted reproduction stems from the principle that people should be free to act as they choose. Moreover, a health carer, at least in a general sense, might well share this belief. Mrs S, it might be said, has the right to a real choice about whether to have a child or not.

It is generally agreed that there is more than one sort of right. Legal rights, for instance, are those that have been enshrined in law; moral rights may not have legal expression, but may be widely acknowledged in a society (individual freedom is widely valued in some countries). Other rights are claimed, but disputed, for instance the 'right' to abortion in some States. One thing that differentiates among 'rights' is whether or not they can be said to entail some obligation or duty upon others to make sure they are realised. If Mrs S's right to assisted conception is of the strength that does establish an obligation, then some reciprocal duty devolves upon relevant institutions and people in them.

No legal right to assisted conception currently exists, but there may be an argument for its being an acknowledged moral right. Whether such an argument is compelling will depend on the basis of the right itself. A claim to assisted conception might be built upon arguments from justice, or from the distress which results from being childless. But would either foundation be sufficient to be the basis of an undoubted moral right to assisted conception?

For Mrs S, being without a child may be the cause of serious unhappiness. It may even be a temptation to describe having a child as a need for her. Certainly it is a matter of great distress for some that they are childless. The possibility arises that this distress is in some cases so sharp as to give rise to a health concern that may translate into an overriding obligation to respond to it and alleviate it.

But the mere existence of distress does not establish an irrefutable duty to relieve it. Suppose a person wanted a child simply in order to satisfy with the child some deeply felt sexual urge. This desire might be so strongly felt as to be accounted distressing if not met. But desires such as this would be vigorously and publicly condemned. Strong desires are subject to public moral assessment, and as such cannot always and everywhere establish a duty on others to respond by helping to meet them, however distressing or painful it might be for someone not to have her desires met.

Health carers may well be the agents of such public moral assessment—although they need not be the only sources of them. So, despite the fact that Mrs S, or Ms J, is distressed (although not for the reason suggested above) a health carer may still take into account the interests of the child, and on that basis could justifiably refuse assisted reproduction.

So, an overriding moral duty has not yet been established, and the original assertion remains tenable. However, it was suggested previously that rights might be based on fairness or justice. Someone who could not have a child in the usual way might say that they had a right to a child nonetheless, on the grounds that it was unfair that others could have children while she could not. Such considerations of fairness or justice could constitute a compelling moral argument that health carers must respond so as to help those who request aid.

An argument from fairness, justice or equality may be a stronger one than that from distress. This is because it can claim equality in two aspects: first of opportunity (to have a child) and second of treatment (as a parent like any other parent).

As to the first, on its own it is in fact no stronger a claim than that from rights or that from distress. While it is a moral argument in favour of helping Mrs S to conceive, it does not obviate the interests of the child, and perhaps justify acting upon them so as to deny help to her. For instance, the risk of the child being so severely handicapped that its life would be unremittingly awful might justify refusal to offer Mrs S the opportunity to bear a child genetically related to her.

It is here that Mrs S might seem to have recourse to the second aspect of equality, by arguing that she is being treated quite differently from other prospective parents, in that health carers are being allowed to interfere with her choices. She might say that as the interests of the child do not justify such social interference to prevent normal unassisted conception, those same interests should not operate to prevent assisted conception either.

But there is a problem with this argument. In claiming on the grounds of justice that society should not interfere with the lives of those who are unable to have a child (except by assisted conception) any more than it interferes in the lives of those who do not need medical help to conceive, Mrs S seems to undermine her claim to help from an infertility clinic. After all, that too is an interference, although some may prefer to call it an intervention. In other words, the two forms of intervention are applied unequally. What differentiates them is whether or not people think they are morally good interventions. Mrs S, or Ms J, may value the medical intervention, and disvalue the social interference; but others may value the intervention to protect the interests of the possible child. Society may, on the whole, value both interventions, sometimes preferring the former, most often applying both, but just occasionally choosing the latter where it contradicts the former.

But this conclusion seems to take for granted that society may intervene where it chooses, and whether it may has yet to be shown. Ms J may request society's help to conceive: is that justification for society to do anything other than she requests it to do? One answer may be this: society always has an obligation to children, but under normal circumstances that obligation before conception is overridden by other obligations (for instance, to uphold the privacy of its citizens). Where circumstances are such that people have to involve society in a usually private choice, it does not follow that society should waive other obligations (for instance to the child).

Thus the second objection to the assertion that the interests of the child may on occasion justify refusing to treat the infertile falls: no unavoidable moral duty to treat those requesting infertility treatment emerges. The assertion seems now to have some strength, having survived the argument that no moral judgements can be made (since they can be), and the immediately following argument that there are unavoidable duties to help the infertile, established by rights, distress or justice (since there are not).

Infertility is (morally) a disease like any other

In asserting that the interests of the child might provide justification for refusing treatment to Mrs S or Ms J, it was argued that health carers working in infertility treatment have some responsibility to the child which might result from their helping an infertile woman or couple. The existence of this responsibility was said to allow the possibility that the interests of the child could override any duty or desire to help couples wanting a baby.

However, perhaps there is a mistake here. Possibly, while the interests of the child may quite rightly be considered, in the final analysis those interests must be secondary to the duty of the health carer to treat the infertility of her patient. For, in the end, it may be argued that infertility is, in general and in moral terms, a disease like any other, and that for that reason the primary responsibility of the health carer is to the client or patient who is infertile.

The claim here is not that infertility is like cancer (life-threatening) or like rheumatoid arthritis (debilitating and painful). The point of similarity is not in the particular symptoms, physiological effects or pathology, but rather in the fact that infertility is by its very nature just another disease. It has symptoms, physiological ramifications and pathology. And what is said to follow from this is that those like Ms J, or any others, who may be said to 'suffer' from infertility, should be treated as they would be had they got pneumonia. (Mrs S may fall outside this category, as she is not apparently infertile.)

If this argument holds it would seem to establish that, at least where infertility is the cause of childlessness, the choices that those who are infertile make once infertility is circumvented should ultimately be up to them. Health carers, then, may appropriately or otherwise advise Ms J that a child requires a stable home background and exhort her to marry one of her partners in the interests of her baby, but not refuse to help her overcome her infertility if she refuses to alter her lifestyle.

This conclusion is plausible so long as infertility is a disease, and is morally like any other disease. Whether infertility is a disease rests upon what 'disease' means. This is an issue that has exercised philosophers and doctors, but no agreed definition has emerged (or is likely to emerge). 'Infertility' seems to have fallen into the hands of the health carers, in being defined as a medical problem. However, some clients (and Mrs S may be one) seek assisted conception because they are socially (not clinically) unable to have children. The following arguments do not relate to such people since *prima facie* they are not clinically infertile.

The definition of (clinical) infertility is the inability to conceive a child in the course of 1 year of trying to do so. If this is correct, and conceiving a child is what matters, then it looks as if 'infertility' may indeed be a disease like any other. At the same time, however, the definition seems to call into doubt that infertility is the problem assisted reproduction is intended to treat. Surely, the ultimate problem for Ms J is not that she cannot conceive, but that she is unable (except through assisted conception) to have her own child.

If this seems mistaken, consider a case in which a couple comes to an infertility unit for help to conceive, where the woman is incapable of carrying a child to term. If the clinic can make no provision for surrogacy, would it be sensible to treat her, say with *in vitro* fertilisation (IVF), or with tubal surgery? In fact, it seems to be a pointless thing to do even though it might enable her to conceive. What seems really to matter is that the woman should have a child.

If follows from this point that infertility cannot morally be just like any other disease, thus undermining the objection. Infertility is important because it is a cause of unwanted childlessness for which the only 'cure' is a child (and how odd it sounds to refer to a child in those terms), whose interests may be paramount, and may consist (prior to conception) in not being conceived.

In this second section to the chapter it has been asserted that the interests of a possible child should always arise, and that they may on occasion be decisive in justifying (possibly) a refusal to treat someone who requests assisted reproduction. Thus far, the assertion has been tested by three objections, found to survive all three, and it is somewhat the stronger for doing so.

INTERESTS OTHER THAN THOSE OF THE CHILD

If there is one justification for overriding the claims of the childless couple and on occasions refusing them help to conceive, there may be others. For, in addition to the child's interests there are others that could override those of an infertile person or couple. In the third section of this chapter, I will suggest that in other situations the interests of certain other patients may provide an example of just such another paramount concern.

Suppose a surgeon in obstetrics and gynaecology looks at how her time is parcelled out among her patients. The principal pressures upon her may be the numbers of patients requesting different kinds of help—perhaps she has waiting lists for laparoscopies, hysterectomies and prolapse operations. At the same time, she may already be working as many hours as she reasonably can, so that any increase in time spent on one group of patients must reduce the time she spends with another group.

In this case two ingredients absent from previous examples are now present. They are, first, that there is only a certain amount of time each week and, second, that there are other patients who could use the help of the surgeon. The first added ingredient is obvious enough, but it provides the condition in which the second ingredient takes on its moral significance. For these other people, like the child, and, of course, like the clients for assisted conception, have interests that are morally significant. And they may well have needs, rights or claims of justice that could place duties upon the surgeon. But because time is limited, she will have to choose between these patients.

Time is just one resource that may be limited; money, human skills, machines, space, and many others can also be counted as resources none of which are in endless supply. Any such resource limitation may mean that choices have to be made about where the available resources should be directed. And making such choices among those who may have desires, needs, rights or claims is making a choice with an unavoidable moral dimension to it.

The moral dimension arises thus: suppose the surgeon decides to extend the time she spends doing laparoscopies at the expense of prolapse operations. As a result, these women will have to wait longer than they do already, suffering in consequence a greater period of discomfort and perhaps worry before their surgery, and so on. In increasing her work with those who suffer from childlessness, there are costs of human unhappiness among prolapse patients.

These costs may not be regarded as too high to pay (even by the women who are waiting for prolapse operations). However, some costs may be regarded as too high by almost everybody. For instance, if the choice were to reduce the time spent on hysterectomies, then deaths might result. As against this, the costs of the surgeon not increasing the time spent on assisted conception in her weekly timetable might be that a number of people would never be offered help to conceive at all, or that couples would be limited as to the number of treatment cycles of (say) IVF.

Thus, a restriction in resources (or an increase in demand) will mean that the reasons for which assisted conception is (in effect) refused may have to be extended. For instance, the clinical indications for which certain opportunities are offered may need to be limited. The clinical indications against offering Ms J or anyone else gamete intra-Fallopian transfer (GIFT), for instance, may need to be re-evaluated. But the reason now would not be that (say) GIFT was simply medically inappropriate, but rather that quite proper concerns for other patients made certain kinds of resource expenditure morally unacceptable (in this case, for instance, expense on treatments with less than a certain percentage chance of success). In this way, clinical indications may themselves become morally evaluated, a low rate of success being morally significant.

The same kind of point is sometimes made in other areas of therapy, for instance in the case of provision of intensive care beds, and particularly their use for patients who have suffered heart attacks and have had to be resuscitated. The recovery rate of those who suffer cardiopulmonary arrest and are resuscitated and then taken to the intensive care unit is reputedly very poor. In the mean time, they take up beds that might be used for others with conditions (perhaps less serious) known to benefit more uniformly from intensive care. Perhaps, ideally, all patients who might benefit from intensive care should be offered it. Short of that ideal situation the indications for which patients are sent to intensive care may need to be evaluated, and moral choices made about which costs are acceptable. (Among the complicating factors involved in making such a choice might be this question: is ability to benefit or need the more compelling justification for treatment?)

Certain clinical indications for assisted conception may become the subject of moral assessment in a situation of limited resources. And it is also possible that *moral* issues previously lacking the weight to be justifications for refusing Mrs S or Ms J treatment could in such circumstances become weighty enough to be justifications for such a refusal. In at least one instance it seems that they may. In times of plenty Mrs S's claim might after all be met. Where resources are lacking, however, the claims of all patients might be subject to a different assessment. What may force a decision not to treat Mrs S on to health carers is the relative urgency of other claims, or the greater suffering of others. In short, in an ideal situation, Mrs S's claim might be subject to assessment only in its own right, but in the real world it may also have to be assessed comparatively.

CONCLUSION

It was asserted above that there may be times when the interests of a potential child are contrary to and of greater weight than the interests of a person seeking help to conceive that child. This assertion was tested against three main objections: that it is impossible to make moral judgements of this kind; that there are overriding moral reasons for helping those who seek such help; and that infertility is a disease morally like any other, its circumvention being the prime responsibility of the health carer.

Against these objections, and in favour of the assertion, the chief argument has been that infertility is morally distinct from other diseases. The child is morally significant in its own right. It deserves the concern of health carers, and indeed of others, and in that lies the possibility that a concern for it will outweigh a concern for Mrs S or Ms J. If, then, that concern is met only by the child not being conceived, a justification seems to exist for refusal to treat.

Relevant interests other than those of the child were identified. These may on occasion provide justification for refusing treatment to particular people. Where patients are in competition for resources, whichever patients the health carer chooses to treat, the choice will unavoidably be a moral one between the sufferings, needs, fears and interests of those patients. In such cases the claims of some patients seeking help to conceive may have to be put aside.

What has been said in this chapter may be significant to moral debate about the issue of whether or not to treat some patients who request help to conceive. But it should be emphasised that the arguments here cannot be decisive in isolation from 'life'. For instance, the respective weight given by individuals to the interests of the child and to the interests of the client in any particular situation will vary with the real experiences, and beliefs, of people involved. In their lives, health carers may be struggling with the moral issues mentioned here. Some, after that struggle, may justifiably feel it wrong to treat some of those who ask for assisted conception.

SUGGESTED READING

Book on general moral issues raised in this chapter

Midgely, M. (1991). *Can't We Make Moral Judgements?* Bristol Press, Bristol.

Book with sections on ethical issues in reproductive medicine

Beauchamp, T. L. and Walters, L.–R. (eds) (1982). *Contemporary Issues in Bioethics.* Wadsworth, Belmont, CA.

Books and articles on ethical issues in reproductive medicine

Chadwick, R. F. (ed.) (1990). *Ethics, Reproduction and Genetic Control.* Routledge & Kegan Paul, London.

Council for Science and Society Working Party Report (1984). *Human Procreation: Ethical Aspects of the New Techniques.* Oxford University Press, Oxford.

Glover, J. et al. (1989). *Fertility and the Family. The Glover Report on Reproductive Technologies to the European Commission.* Fourth Estate, London.

Harris, J. (1985). *The Value of Life.* Routledge & Kegan Paul, London.

LaFollette, H. (1980). Licensing parents. *Philos. Public Affairs*, **9**, no. 2.

Lee, R. E. and Morgan, D. (eds) (1990). *Birthrights: Law and Ethics and the Beginning of Life.* Routledge & Kegan Paul, London.

Page, E. (1985). Donation, surrogacy and adoption. *J. Appl. Philos.*, **2**, no. 2.

Singer, P. and Wells, D. (1984). *The Reproduction Revolution: New Ways of Making Babies.* Oxford University Press, Oxford.

Warnock, M. et al. (1985). *A Question of Life: The Warnock Report on Human Fertilisation and Embryology.* Basil Blackwell, Oxford.

8

Pre-menstrual Syndrome

Michael M. Dooley

West Dorset Hospital, Dorchester, UK

Despite the abundance of theories, pre-menstrual syndrome (PMS) is a mystery.

This probably sums up any review of PMS, with persistent conflict as to the existence of the syndrome, a question as to whether it is one syndrome or several, and a debate as to whether the origin is psychic, somatic or both. It is strange that when one considers how many women suffer from this complaint more precise knowledge as to the extent of the problem is not available.

HISTORY

> Many a young life is battered and forever crippled in the breakers of puberty; if it crosses these unharmed and is not dashed to pieces on the rock of childbirth it may still ground on the ever recurring shallows of menstruation and lastly, upon the final bar of the menopause where protection is found in the unruffled waters of the harbour beyond the reach of sexual storms.

The above statement by the President of the American Gynaecological Society in 1900 highlights the many different bridges which a woman, throughout her lifespan, has to cross.

The problems that are encountered during the reproductive life have been well documented in the literature down through the ages. Ayur Veda, in 1000 BC, reported that women complain of dysmenorrhoea. Hippocrates in 400 BC attributed a pre-menstrual-like syndrome to:

> a woman's agitated blood seeking to escape from the womb.

Understanding Common Disorders in Reproductive Endocrinology. Edited by M.M. Dooley and M.P. Brincat.

In 1847 De Wees wrote that menstruation:

> rarely fails to be announced by a variety of symptoms of greater or lesser severity or danger.

The French historian, Jules Michelet, explained that for a period of 15–20 days out of 28 a woman was:

> not only an invalid but a wounded one.

Although much has been written about cyclical menstrual changes in the literature from time immemorial it was not until 1931 that Frank coined the term 'pre-menstrual tension' to describe the distressing symptoms that occur cyclically in women prior to menses.

The term 'pre-menstrual tension' was accepted until 1953 when Green and Dalton stated that the term was unsatisfactory because tension is only one of the many components of the syndrome. In their opinion its use has led to a failure to diagnose the disorder when tension is absent or is overshadowed by another complaint. In view of this they proposed the term 'pre-menstrual syndrome' although they did realise that the term was not totally satisfactory.

The term 'ovarian cycle syndrome' may be more satisfactory as this indicates that the pathology is within the ovary and may occur after a hysterectomy.

DEFINITION

There is an ongoing debate about the definition of PMS. Having reviewed the literature the most comprehensive definition is:

> Premenstrual syndrome is the occurrence of distressing physical and/or psychological symptoms, that interfere with social or work related activities, not caused by any recognisable organic or psychiatric disease, which occur in the luteal phase of the menstrual cycle, improve with menses and disappear completely prior to the next onset of symptoms of premenstrual syndrome.

SYMPTOMS

> It is like being on drugs . . . I feel completely out of control.

explains one woman of her experiences with PMS.

Table 1 Common symptoms of PMS

Emotional and behavioural	
Sadness	Decreased concentration
Anxiety	Indecision
Depression	Paranoia
Irritability	Loss of control
Labile mood	Insomnia
Anorexia	Craving for certain foods
Fatigue	Lethargy
Agitation	Change in libido
Dizzy spells	Clumsiness
Physical	
Headache	Breast tenderness
Joint and muscle pain	Breast swelling
Backache	Acne
Swelling	Gastrointestinal disturbances

It is the timing and severity of the symptoms which are important, and a wide variety of symptoms both somatic and psychological have been related to the menstrual cycle, with up to 150 different symptoms being linked to the menstrual cycle.

There is an extraordinary diversity of symptoms that can occur. These include many of the most common symptoms of each medical specialty and it appears that no tissue in the body is exempt from inclusion. Table 1 lists the common symptoms of PMS.

There is perhaps not one but several subgroups of PMS and indeed each may possibly have its own aetiology and thus require different therapy.

These subgroups could include:

PMS–A: consisting of anxiety, irritability and nervous tension.

PMS–B: symptoms associated with water and salt retention, abdominal bloating, mastalgia and weight control.

PMS–C: associated with pre-menstrual craving for sweets, increased appetite and indulgence in eating refined sugar followed by palpitation, fatigue, fainting spells, headache and sometimes the shakes.

PMS–D: symptoms of depression, withdrawal, insomnia, forgetfulness and confusion.

It could therefore be stated that instead of 'pre-menstrual syndrome' it should be renamed the 'pre-menstrual syndromes'.

PREVALANCE

PMS has been described as the most common of minor endocrine disorders and is one of the most common diseases.

Most women experience some pre-menstrual symptoms but only 20–40% suffer emotional, behavioural and/or physical symptoms severe enough to seek help from their doctors, and in 2–6% of women symptoms are felt to be incapacitating.

The true prevalence is difficult to assess and is obviously dependent on the definition used in the survey and the population surveyed. It is possible that some bias in these analyses may result from the fact that women who suffer from PMS are more likely to be motivated to enter studies or to answer questionnaires when compared to women who are symptomless.

The prevalence of PMS increases after the birth of the first child, and up to 30% of patients note that their problem started with the return of menstruation after the birth of a baby.

There also appears to be an association with post-natal depression, and up to 40% of PMS sufferers have a history of post-partum depression, the normal incidence in the population as a whole being around 10%.

DIAGNOSIS

The approach to diagnosis, as in any other area of medicine, needs to follow the conventional pattern of history, examination and investigation.

History

The diagnosis of PMS depends on the timing of the symptoms in relation to menstruation. Symptoms typically begin in mid-cycle and increase in number and severity to maximum intensity the day before or at the onset of bleeding.

At the first consultation care must be taken as up to 50% of women claiming to have PMS do not have this confirmed following daily menstrual charting in a prospective manner. Prior to any treatment it is useful to have at least 1 month's untreated daily scoring as a baseline.

There are some indicators in the history which are important to determine whether present. These include a history of post-natal depression which, as already stated, occurs in 40% of cases. Pre-menstrual symptoms are absent during pregnancy and it has been stated that PMS sufferers feel unusually well after the first trimester.

Contraceptive history can be informative, as being on the oral contraceptive pill reduces the symptoms.

Questioning should also be directed towards diet as not only may some women develop pre-menstrual cravings, especially for glucose, but a high salt intake may predispose to PMS.

Examination

Examination is essential in all PMS sufferers, not only for the positive but also for the negative findings and in order to help exclude other pathology.

A general examination including weight, blood pressure and breast examination is useful to have as a baseline for treatment. A vaginal examination will help to exclude gross gynaecological abnormality including fibroids, ovarian cysts and endometriosis.

Investigations

Routine blood investigations are of limited value.

If the woman is sexually active then a routine cervical smear, if not previously performed, should be performed at this opportune moment.

Questionnaires

A menstrual calendar is helpful in the diagnosis of PMS as often the diagnosis is erroneously made. Several different calendars/questionnaires/forms have been proposed and each have limitations.

Simple questionnaires are of benefit for routine clinical assessment of PMS but may not be valid for research. Such charts can be seen in Figure 1.

A diagnostic disc has been developed, the PMT-cator, which allows women to score their symptoms throughout their cycle and by using a simple calculation assess if they have a significant degree of pre-menstrual distress. This has been devised at the PMT Clinic, Dulwich Hospital, London (see Figure 2).

To date no ideal method of diagnosis has been demonstrated. A simple reliable questionnaire, which does not require too much commitment from the patient, is prospective rather than retrospective, which allows an objective method for reliable diagnosis and ideally monitoring the treatment and provides material for statistical analysis is urgently needed, although the PMT-cator does go some way towards answering these questions.

Name ______________________

Address ______________________

Date ______________

LMP ______________

Day / Month	1	2	3	4	5	6	7	8	9	10	11	12	13	14	15	16	17	18	19	20	21	22	23	24	25	26	27	28	29	30	31	**TOTAL**

Please fill in the chart to help aid the diagnosis of premenstrual syndrome. **Bleeding** should be documented by the letter b in the appropriate boxes. If you could then write down below the five important symptoms that you complain of and indicate them against the appropriate number. Please then fill in the chart for the next 3 months.

Important symptoms

1
2
3
4
5

Figure 1 A simple questionnaire for PMS

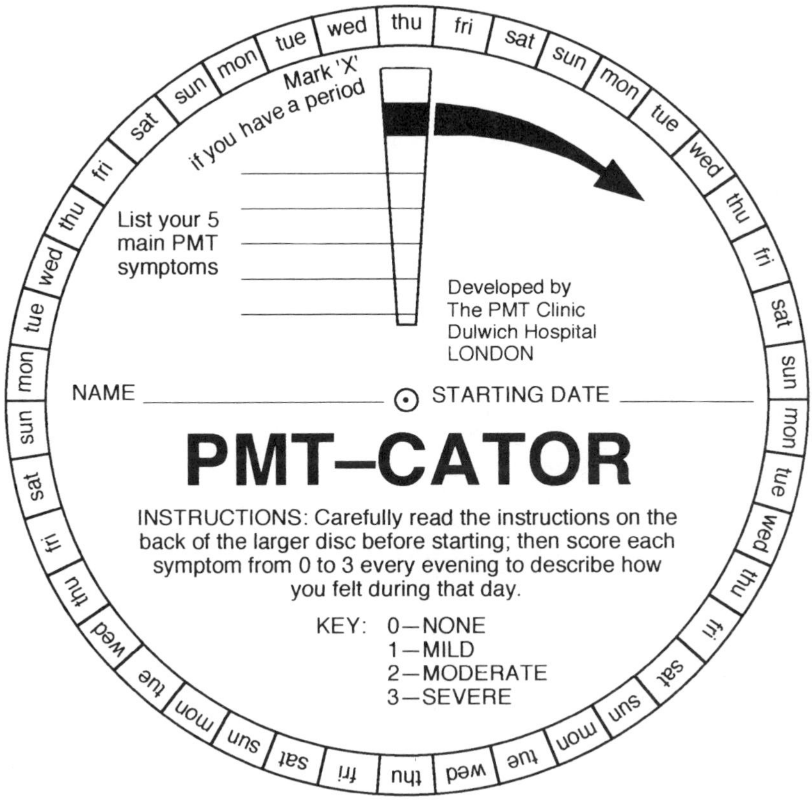

Figure 2 A diagnostic 'PMT-cator' enabling patients to score symptoms throughout a cycle. This is available from Rocket of London, Imperial Way, Watford. Reproduced from Magos and Studd, 1984, by permission of Churchill Livingstone

PATHOPHYSIOLOGY

Very little is understood about the pathophysiology of the syndrome and there is much speculation. This is perhaps the core of the confusion which exists in the areas of PMS. If agreement could be reached as to the pathophysiology then criteria for diagnosis, correct syndrome name and proper treatment would quickly follow. Enthusiastic investigators in this field often throw up anecdotal pieces of evidence and try and base firm aetiological explanations on these flimsy bits of information. Sadly this often adds more to the discredit of PMS.

The primary pathology is within the ovary. Prior to puberty, during pregnancy and in post-menopausal women PMS does not occur. Oophorectomy will also prevent PMS. Any pathophysiological process must therefore take this into account and to date no exact mechanism for the development of PMS has been formulated.

The different postulated pathophysiological mechanisms include:

- Oestrogen:progesterone imbalance.
- Vitamin B6 deficiency.
- Vitamin A deficiency.
- Prolactin imbalance.
- Essential fatty acid and prostaglandin imbalance.
- Upset in the renin–angiotensin–aldosterone system.
- Deficiency in sex hormone-binding globulin capacity.
- Endogenous hormone allergy.
- Hypoglycaemia.
- Psychogenic.

Confusion certainly exists with regard to the aetiology.

Argument is followed by counter-argument. As new treatments arrive and biochemical tests are developed, another aetiology for PMS is presenting. There is probably not one cause as there probably is not one syndrome. Equally there is no one treatment. Environmental factors play a role in the aetiology as do endocrine factors. The neuroendocrine system is only now beginning to be fully understood. Perhaps PMS is a multifactorial psychoneuroendocrine disorder.

TREATMENT

Any treatment regimes and especially clinical trials for PMS are always shadowed by the high placebo response, up to 80%, that this syndrome demonstrates.

Prior to any pharmacological treatment advice on a healthy diet, adequate exercise and education on the actual syndrome are all important. A sympathetic clear explanation of why they are experiencing symptoms, coupled with reassurance that these symptoms are part of a normal cycle and no serious organic disease process, is all-important.

Patient support

The key to any successful treatment is careful assessment and strong positive reassurance. In all cases it is important for the doctor to have a sympathetic approach, reassure the patient that she is not unique and explain the nature of any treatment.

'Pre-menstrual complainers' may be high-stress subjects, and the management and alleviation of stress is of importance in the practical management of women with PMS.

Dietary advice

Maintaining steady blood glucose levels may benefit women with PMS, and changing to a 3-hourly starch diet may help to relieve symptoms.

Vitamin B6

Pyridoxine (vitamin B6) has been used for many years in doses of 50–300 mg per day. To date few studies using vitamin treatment of PMS have involved placebo controls, and many studies are methodologically flawed. Doses exceeding 2 g daily can be dangerous and may cause serious neuropathy.

Bromocriptine

As already indicated, prolactin has been implicated in the pathophysiology of PMS. Doses of bromocriptine up to 2.5 mg twice daily reduce cyclical breast pain and may improve other symptoms, including headache, mood changes and bloatedness.

Evening primrose oil (gamolenic acid)

This may be useful for a wide variety of symptoms associated with PMS. It has been postulated that some women have reduced levels of essential fatty acids which can be corrected by the use of evening primrose oil. The dose required needs to be high in order to get adequate absorption.

Prostaglandin synthase inhibitors

Mefenamic acid in doses up to 250 mg three times a day starting 12 days before the anticipated onset of menstruation, increasing to 500 mg three times a day from 9 days pre-menstrually, has been demonstrated to improve fatigue, headache, general aches and pains and mood swings.

Progesterone

Dalton, as documented in her book *Premenstrual Syndrome and Progesterone Therapy*, has used progesterone for nearly 30 years in the treatment of PMS.

She feels that failure of patients with PMS to respond is due either to incorrect diagnosis or incorrect frequency or dosage of progesterone. The efficacy of natural progesterone treatment appears to be at a pharmacological level rather than simply making up any deficiency and thus improve the progesterone–oestradiol ratio. There is no consistent evidence that progesterone levels are altered in women with PMS.

Several well-controlled placebo studies have failed to demonstrate significant improvement with PMS by the use of progesterone in doses up to 800 mg per day.

Progestagens

Many different progestagens have been studied. Different progestagens have very varied actions and some may promote symptoms of PMS of their own. Indeed, norethisterone has powerful water-retaining characteristics. Again no well-controlled studies demonstrate benefit of progestagens over a placebo in the treatment of PMS.

Oral contraceptive

The report of the Royal College of General Practitioners (1974) recorded the incidence of PMS to be 29% less in 'pill' takers than 'non-pill' users. Oral contraceptives are useful drugs in the treatment of PMS. Some women develop PMS symptoms in the 'pill-free' week and it has been suggested that this may be overcome by continuous therapy if the woman is prepared to accept erratic or absent periods.

Oestrogen

Oestrogens have been used with the aim to suppress ovulation and thus suppress cyclical ovarian activity. Such regimes, including oestradiol implants or transdermal oestradiol patches, appear very successful. Concomitant treatment with cyclical progestagen for up to 12 days of each cycle will prevent endometrial hyperplasia.

Luteinising hormone-releasing hormone

Muse et al. (1984) reported a cross-over study, conducted over a 6-month period, in eight patients with well-characterised PMS in which physical behavioural symptoms were relieved by daily administration of an agonist of gonadotrophin-releasing hormone. They were very quick to indicate that such treatment would not be long-term because of the increased risk of osteoporosis. It may be useful in aiding the diagnosis of the syndrome.

Danazol

Danazol, which suppresses gonadotrophin stimulation and abolishes cyclical ovarian function, has a role in the treatment of PMS. In low doses (200 mg per day) danazol may be of benefit in PMS. In the larger doses that induce amenorrhoea side-effects, including acne, may be unacceptable.

Placebo effects

The placebo aspect appears to be an effective part of the treatment. Severe symptoms may not be completely improved but their severity is often dramatically reduced.

The mere fact that a patient discusses the problem with her doctor and receives sympathetic support may well cause the stress factor to be relieved and even the physiology at the hypothalamic level to return to normal.

CONCLUSION

PMS is common and can significantly disrupt the life of many women. No one knows the basic cause(s) of PMS but almost every doctor has at least one favourite treatment.

Explanation and reassurance is all-important, especially when the high placebo response is taken into consideration.

Many different pharmacological and dietary agents are available for treatment and as one may be dealing with a variety of different aetiologies it may be necessary to try different treatment regimes in order to find the most suitable one for a particular patient.

SUGGESTED READING

Dalton, K. (1984). *The Premenstrual Syndrome and Progesterone Therapy* (2nd edn). Heinemann, London.

Magos, A. and Studd, J. (1984). The premenstrual syndrome. In *Progress in Obstetrics and Gynaecology* (Vol. 4). Churchill Livingstone, Edinburgh.

Magos, A. L., Brincat, M. and Studd, J. W. W. (1986). Treatment of premenstrual syndrome by subcutaneous implants and cyclical oral norethisterone: placebo controlled study. *Br. Med. J.*, **292**, 1629–1633.

Managing the premenstrual syndrome (1992). *Drugs Ther. Bull.*, **30**, 69–72.

Muse, K. N. (1989). Clinical experience with the use of GnRH agonists in the treatment of premenstrual syndrome. *Obstet. Gynecol. Surv.*, **44**, 317–318.

Royal College of General Practitioners (1974). *Oral Contraceptives and Health.* Pitman Medical, London.

Watson, N. R., Savvas, M., Studd, J. W. W., Garnett, T. and Baber, R. J. (1989). Treatment of severe premenstrual syndrome with oestradiol patches and cyclical oral norethisterone. *Lancet*, **ii**, 730–732.

9

Hormonal Contraception

P. G. Crosignani* and C. La Vecchia†
*University of Milan and †Mario Negri Institute, Milan, Italy

COMBINATION PILL

Pharmacology

The combination oral contraceptives contain various doses of two synthetic oestrogens, ethinyl oestradiol or ethinyl oestradiol-3-methyl ether (mestranol), and of 10 different progestins. There are many different combination oral contraceptive formulations available for use.

Oestrogen

All combination oral contraceptives contain ethinyl oestradiol or its 3-methyl ether, mestranol. Mestranol must be converted to ethinyl oestradiol to be biologically active (Kappus and Remmer, 1973). In various bioassays, mestranol appears to have approximately 30% less bioactivity than ethinyl oestradiol (Delforge and Ferin, 1970).

Serum levels of ethinyl oestradiol peak approximately 1 h after oral ingestion, fall rapidly for 6 h and then decline slowly. Ingestion of mestranol results in peak serum ethinyl oestradiol concentrations approximately 2–4 h after oral ingestion (De la Pena et al., 1975). Twenty-four hours after the oral administration of ethinyl oestradiol, approximately one third of the drug appears in the urine as glucuronide conjugates, one third is excreted into the faeces, and one third is still in the circulation (Reed et al., 1972). The ethinyl oestradiol conjugates excreted into the bowel can be hydrolysed by enteric bacteria and re-enter the circulation. Drugs that alter enteric flora (e.g. antibiotics) can alter this enterohepatic circulation and result in increased faecal

Understanding Common Disorders in Reproductive Endocrinology. Edited by M.M. Dooley and M.P. Brincat.

excretion of ethinyl oestradiol, which may, in some instances, result in a failure of the oral contraceptive to suppress ovulation (Adlercreutz et al., 1979).

Progestagen

All progestins but one (cyproterone acetate) are 19-nortestosterone derivatives; they are norethindrone, norethindrone acetate, norethynodrel, norgestrel, ethynodiol diacetate, desogestrel and gestodene norgestimate.

The initial step in the action of any steroid hormone is interaction of the steroid with an intranuclear steroid receptor. Many synthetic progestins bind to several classes of receptors. For example, norethindrone binds well to progesterone and androgen receptors, and one of its metabolites binds to oestrogen receptors (Larrea et al., 1987). Consequently, norethindrone has progestational, oestrogenic and androgenic effects *in vivo*. The androgenic properties of the synthetic progestins have important clinical consequences on lipid and carbohydrate metabolism.

There is a peak approximately 1.5–3 h after oral ingestion of progestagen and at 24 h values in the serum are still between 20% and 25% of the original peak. After 5 days of use, norgestrel is still detectable for 5 days after discontinuation of therapy (Brenner et al., 1977). These levels are sufficient to suppress gonadotrophins for 4–6 days after the last pill was ingested.

Mechanism of action

Combination oral contraceptives produce multiple effects on the reproductive system. Of all these effects, the most important is their suppression of the hypothalamic–pituitary system. The mid-cycle surge of gonadotrophins is consistently inhibited, thus blocking ovulation. The exogenous hormone renders cervical mucus thick and scanty, which retards sperm penetration. Combination oral contraceptives alter uterine and tubal motility. The production of glycogen by the endometrial glands is diminished by the ingestion of oral contraceptives, and this impairs survival of the blastocyst in the uterine cavity. They also alter the ovarian response to gonadotrophin stimulation.

The first pill of each cycle is the most important one not to miss, because it is taken after 7 days of no steroid intake. When a patient misses one pill, she should take it the next day in addition to that day's pill. When the patient misses two consecutive pills, there is a much greater chance of breakthrough ovulation (Morris et al., 1979; Chowdhury et al., 1980).

Oral contraceptives are the most effective form of reversible contraception. Effectiveness is usually spoken of as method or use effectiveness. Many factors of patient compliance influence use effectiveness. When used properly, a contraceptive's use effectiveness can approach its theoretical method effectiveness. From a study of a very motivated population, Vessey and others reported a failure rate of 0.3 per 100 women-years. In another study, Grady et al. found failure rates per 100 women-years to be 2.9 for the pill, 6.0 for intrauterine contraceptive device (IUCD), 14.1 for condom, 17.2 for the diaphragm, and 16.1 for the rhythm method (Grady et al., 1986).

Metabolic effects

Oral contraceptives produce other metabolic alterations besides changes in the reproductive axis (European Consensus Committee, 1990). Some metabolic changes are related to the dose of the oestrogen component and some are related to the dose of the progestin component (Table 1). All currently used oral contraceptives can cause deterioration in glucose tolerance, accompanied by hyperinsulinaemia. The magnitude of the impact on glucose metabolism depends mainly on the type of progestagen and also on the dose of a given steroid. The changes in lipid and lipoprotein metabolism induced by oral contraceptives are also dose-dependent and related to both oestrogens and progestagens. The progestagen component is mainly responsible for the effects of oral contraceptives on metabolism, but the oestrogen component may modulate the influence. Oral contraceptives alter haemostatic variables, although usually not beyond the normal range. A number of studies have shown changes in the coagulation system indicative of increased activation and in the fibrolytic system of increased reaction product concentrations. It is conceivable that these effects are oestrogen-mediated, because they have not been demonstrated in progestagen-only preparations. For oestrogens there is a dose-dependent relationship, although in the combination pills the progestagens might have modifying effects.

Oral contraceptive formulations containing 30–35 μg of ethinyl oestradiol per tablet are associated with very low pregnancy rates (similar to formulations with higher doses of oestrogen) and have negligible metabolic effects. The use of oestrogen-containing formulations with less than 50 μg of oestrogen had steadily increased, to nearly 90% of all European prescriptions in 1989. Therefore routine screening of all oral contraceptive users for altered carbohydrate metabolism is not recommended, although it is still desirable, but it should not preclude their use in women who have high-risk factors for deterioration of carbohydrate metabolism, such as gestational diabetes, obesity or first-degree relatives with diabetes. There is no evidence that the lipid changes are related to atherogenesis in oral contraceptive users, but it is prudent to prescribe an oral contraceptive with minimal effects on lipids. In women with a suggestive family history for thrombophilia (deficiency in antithrombin III, protein S or protein C), the risk, may be exacerbated by oral contraceptive use and the present diagnostic possibilities for detecting risk of cardiovascular diseases provide very little useful information.

Table 1 Metabolic effects of oestrogen and progestagen

Affected substance or function	Effect	Clinical significance
OESTROGEN		
Proteins		
Albumin	–	None
Globulins	+	
Angiotensinogen		↑ Blood pressure
Clotting factors I, VII, X		Hypercoagulation
Carrier proteins		None
Lipids		
Cholesterol	=	None
Triglycerides	+	None
HDL cholesterol	+	↓ Vascular risk
LDL cholesterol	–	↓ Vascular risk
Electrolytes		
Sodium excretion	+	Fluid retention
Tryptophan metabolism	–	Depression
Skin		
Sebum production	–	↓ Acne
Pigmentation	+	Chloasma
PROGESTAGEN		
Carbohydrates		
Plasma insulin	+	None
Glucose tolerance	–	None
Lipids		
Cholesterol	–	None
Triglycerides	–	None
HDL cholesterol	–	↑ Vascular risk
LDL cholesterol	+	↑ Vascular risk
Nitrogen retention	+	↑ Body weight
Skin		
Sebum production	+	↑ Acne

Oral contraceptive use may also alter standard laboratory tests via the mechanisms noted above (Miale and Kent, 1974).

Drug interactions

When oral contraceptive users take other medications concomitantly, there is a risk of decreased effectiveness of the oral contraceptive or of alterations of the effectiveness of the other medication (Wah and Barbieri, 1988). The new low-dose formulations have a smaller margin for variation of the serum levels of steroids needed to suppress ovulation and be effective in contraception (Diczfalusy, 1986). One of the most significant interactions is between oral contraceptives and rifampicin (Back et al., 1980), a potent inducer of liver enzymes. This induction of hepatic enzymes leads to increased metabolism of the steroids in the oral contraceptives. This leads to a decrease in the serum levels of the oral contraceptive steroids, which may allow ovulation from decreased gonadotrophin suppression. A less serious sign of interaction is breakthrough bleeding. Evaluation of breakthrough bleeding must include a careful inquiry about other medications used concomitantly with oral contraceptives. Table 2 summarises the interactions between medications and oral contraceptives.

Non-contraceptive benefits of oral contraceptive use

The considerable non-contraceptive health benefits associated with oral contraceptive use are not well known to either the consumer or the contraceptive counsellor. The benefits of consistent inhibition of ovulation by contraceptives include lowered incidences of functional ovarian cysts, ovarian cancer, benign breast disease, dysmenorrhoea and PMS. The benefits due to inhibition of synthesis of oestrogen receptors by the synthetic progestin are reduced incidences of endometrial cancer, and regulation of menstrual blood loss. Another non-contraceptive health benefit of birth control pill use is a 50% decrease in the risk of acute salpingitis as compared with a control group using no method of contraception. Furthermore oral contraceptive use protects against ectopic pregnancy. Oestrogens decrease and gestagens increase sebum production. Patients who have acne may benefit from an oestrogen-dominant formulation.

Symptoms associated with the use of oral contraceptives

The symptoms produced by the oestrogen component are nausea, breast tenderness and fluid retention. Symptoms produced by the progestin component include weight gain, acne, amenorrhoea and possibly nervousness.

Progestins suppress endometrial growth, and consequently some women do not have withdrawal bleeding. Although amenorrhoea during oral contraception is not of medical significance, it removes the monthly signal that is reassuring to the woman. Breakthrough bleeding and chloasma are adverse effects that are attributed to both components of the pill. Breakthrough bleeding results from too little oestrogen or too much progestin, or both. Almost all of these adverse effects occur most commonly in the initial oral contraception treatment cycles and tend to disappear with continued birth

Table 2 Phamacological interaction of oral contraceptives

	Mechanism	Interaction degree	Recommendation
Drugs lowering contraceptive effectiveness			
Rifampicin	Induces hepatic microsomal enzymes, increasing oral contraceptive steroid metabolism, destroys bacteria	+++	Use alternative form of contraception
Phenobarbitone	Induces hapatic microsomal enzymes, increasing oral contraceptive steroid metabolism	++	Use higher-dosage oral contraceptive or use alternative form of contraceptive
Phenytoin		++	
Griseofulvin		++	
Ampicillin	Destroys enteric bacteria	+	Use additional form of contraception if breakthrough bleeding occurs
Tetracycline		+	
Drugs affected by concurrent oral contraceptive use			
Dicumarol	Oral contraceptive decreases effectiveness	+++	Concurrent use should be avoided
Troleandomycin	Incidence of cholestatic jaundice	+++	
Imipramine	Decreases hepatic oxidation of imipramine	++	Decreased imipramine dose to two thirds
Prednisolone	Decreases hepatic metabolism of corticosteroids	++	Adjust dosage
Phenobarbitone	Causes fluid retention, which may lower seizure control	+	Monitor for changes in seizure control when oral contraceptive is started or stopped
Phenytoin		+	Look for changes in seizure control
Aminophylline	Inhibits metabolism of aminophylline	+	Adjust dosage
Cyclosporine	Decreases hepatic metabolism and elimination of cyclosporine	+	Monitor hepatic function and cyclosporine levels
Diazepam	Decreases hepatic oxidation of benzodiazepines	+	Monitor plasma levels of diazepines

control pill use. Chloasma is accentuated by sunlight and usually takes a long time to disappear after oral contraceptives are discontinued.

Pregnancy after discontinuation of oral contraceptives

Women using oral contraceptives have a slower rate of return to fertility than women who discontinue other methods of contraception. However, it has been reported that after approximately 2–3 years fertility rates in both users and non-users of oral contraceptives are comparable (Vessey et al., 1976).

There is still concern about the reproductive performance of women after discontinuation of oral contraception. There is no evidence that oral contraception leads to an increased rate of spontaneous abortions or congenital anomalies after discontinuation (Wilson and Brent, 1981). There is a current controversy about the effects of women taking oral contraceptives while unknowingly pregnant. Ingestion of female hormones can lead to abnormal development of genital organs but there is no defined evidence that a therapeutic abortion must be performed if pregnancy is discovered during oral contraceptive use (Vessey et al., 1976).

An increased risk of conceiving monozygotic twins within a year after oral contraceptive use has been reported recently, but the observation needs further confirmation (Murphy et al., 1989).

Contraindications

The US Food and Drug Administration (FDA) label lists the following contraindications to oral contraceptive use:

1. Thrombophlebitis or thromboembolic disorders.
2. Past history of deep vein thrombophlebitis or thromboembolic disorders.
3. Cerebrovascular or coronary artery disease.
4. Known or suspected carcinoma of the breast.
5. Known or suspected oestrogen-dependent neoplasia.
6. Undiagnosed abnormal genital bleeding.
7. Known or suspected pregnancy.
8. A benign or malignant liver tumour that develops during the use of oral contraceptives or other oestrogen-containing medication.

Epidemiology

Oral contraceptives have been investigated more extensively in epidemiological studies than any other class of drugs, and detailed information is now available for most positive or adverse effects of the pill, though there is permanent controversy about a few issues.

Women considering use of oral contraceptives are concerned that the ingestion of the birth control pill will increase their risk of developing cancer or gallbladder disease, adversely affect their potential for future childbearing, and enhance their chance of developing heart attacks and strokes.

Cholelithiasis

The incidence of cholelithiasis is about twice normal for women who have been using oral contraceptives for 4 years or less. The incidence of gallbladder disease decreases to less than normal after approximately 4 years of oral contraceptive use. Thus, oral contraceptive use appears to accelerate the process of cholelithiasis but does not increase its overall incidence. It is not known whether or not the new oral contraceptive formulations that contain less than 50 μg of oestrogen promote the development of gallbladder disease.

Vascular diseases

The relative risk calculated from the three large cohort studies (Royal College of General Practitioners, 1974; Vessey et al., 1976; Ramcharan et al., 1981) was increased about twofold for cardiovascular and cerebrovascular diseases for current oral contraceptive users, and there was a similar increase for ischaemic heart disease mortality.

There now appears to be convincing evidence that the elevated risk is restricted to current users, with no material association observed in ex-users (Stampfer et al., 1988; Rosenberg et al., 1990).

Case–control studies of myocardial infarction (Vessey and Doll, 1968; Mann et al., 1976; Jick et al., 1978; Shapiro et al., 1979), being based on substantially greater numbers of cases, could be used for more detailed analyses of interaction with other risk factors, such as smoking, hypertension or hyperlipidaemia. The overall evidence indicates that the role of oral contraceptives is apparently independent of that of other factors, i.e. multiplicative on the relative risk (RR). Thus, the RR (although not the absolute excess risk) was similar for different age groups. Conversely, the RR calculated from a large multicentre American study (Shapiro et al., 1979) rose to 39 for oral contraceptive users who were heavy smokers as compared to non-smokers or non-oral contraceptive users. Such grossly elevated risk estimates are, clearly, of major concern for women exposed simultaneously to both risk factors but, on the other hand, they offered extremely useful indications for prevention, since avoidance by those women of at least one of the risk factors would substantially reduce the risk. In terms of practical implications for prescription, this indicates that the avoidance of oral contraceptives by women above age 35 or 40 and/or at high risk of ischaemic heart disease for other reasons would avoid, and indeed has avoided (Stadel, 1981), most of the excess risk of cardiovascular diseases associated with oral contraceptives.

These indications for selective prescription, based on earlier epidemiological findings, have probably been even more important, for public health, in reducing vascular risk than the changes in composition (particularly the lower oestrogen content) of newer pills. It is possible, indeed, that the paucity of epidemiological data about the newer pills and cardiovascular events is due, at least in part, to the decreased prevalence of vascular events related to oral contraceptives, and to the consequently greater difficulties of conducting studies of acceptable statistical power.

Breast cancer

Despite the large number of published studies, the debate about the possible association between oral contraceptives and breast cancer is still unsettled. The overall evidence, so far, is reassuring: there is no consistent evidence that breast cancer rates in any age group have been substantially influenced by the widespread use of the oral contraceptives in Western countries. Most case–control and cohort studies, as well as a formal overview (Prentice and Thomas, 1987) based on 16 studies and over 12 000 cases, indicate that breast cancer risk is not higher for users of oral contraceptives than for never-users: the summary RR was 1.0, with a very narrow confidence interval (0.9 to 1.1), and no significant heterogeneity between studies.

There is, however, a subgroup of women for whom a positive association between oral contraceptives and breast cancer has been repeatedly observed: these are younger (i.e. below age 35 or perhaps up to age 45), long-term oral contraceptive users (Lubin et al., 1982; Pike et al., 1983; Rosenberg et al., 1984; Stadel et al., 1985; Meirik et al., 1986; La Vecchia et al., 1986; Paul et al., 1986; McPherson et al., 1987; Ravnihar et al., 1988; Kay and Hannaford, 1988; Miller et al., 1989; Jick et al., 1989; Olsson et al., 1989; Romieu et al., 1989; Stanford et al., 1989). This has led to speculation that long-term use of oral contraceptives at early ages induces unfavourable modifications in the breast, and that the impact of the pill on breast carcinogenesis may become appreciable only after a long 'latent period' and hence that we are now observing only the start of a future pill-induced breast cancer epidemic (McPherson et al., 1986).

In addition to pharmacological and biological considerations, there is, however, direct epidemiological evidence that the effects of oral contraceptives on various female hormone-related neoplasms are similar to those of pregnancy: in fact, the pill lowers the risk of ovarian and endometrial cancer and probably increases that of cervical cancer (see below).

Along this same line, the elevated breast cancer risk for young long-term oral contraceptive users would not necessarily indicate that the same excess risk will be reproduced at later ages. In fact, various hypotheses, including the persistence of these increased risks, their flattening off, or even their reversal in the medium–long term, seem equally reasonable (Bruzzi et al., 1988).

The elucidation of the timing of the relationship of oral contraceptives to breast cancer is, of course, crucial for defining the long-term implications of oral contraceptives for breast cancer risk, and hence ultimately for quantifying any risk–benefit analysis of oral contraceptives and disease. Only future studies, however, will be able to study the long-term impact of early, long-lasting oral contraceptive use, and hence to provide a reliable evaluation of this issue.

Cervical neoplasia

Two cohort studies (Royal College of General Practitioners, 1974; Vessey et al., 1976) and six case–control studies (Thomas, 1972; Ory et al., 1977; Fasal et al., 1981; La Vecchia et al., 1986; Molina et al., 1988; Irwin et al., 1988) have considered dysplasias and *in situ* neoplasias of the cervix uteri. Their results indicate a moderately elevated RR among oral contraceptive users: the overall RR (Prentice and Thomas, 1987) was greater than two (within a lower 95% confidence limit of 1.6) for cohort studies, and although less strongly, still significantly above one (RR = 1.3) for case–control studies as well.

For invasive cervical cancer, most published studies (three cohort studies: Royal College of General Practitioners, 1974; Vessey et al., 1976; Adolsek et al., 1983; and five case–control studies: World Health Organization, 1985; Brinton et al., 1986; La Vecchia et al., 1986; Celentano et al., 1987; Irwin et al., 1988) have found an elevated risk among oral contraceptive users. The overall relative risk estimate was 1.2 for case–control studies, and in two out of three cohort studies all the invasive cancers (13 and six, respectively) were found in pill users.

There is, therefore, consistent evidence indicating that oral contraceptive use is associated with an increased risk of intraepithelial and invasive cervical cancer. This is further confirmed by the precence of direct duration–risk relationships in most studies. Uncertainties concerning cervical neoplasia and oral contraceptives derived chiefly from the potential confounding effects of some important risk correlates, such as sexual habits and, to a lesser extent, smoking, although most recent investigations (La Vecchia et al., 1986; World Health Organization, 1985; Brinton et al., 1986) have attempted to adjust for them.

Since invasive cervical cancer, on the other hand, is largely preventable through rational use of cervical screening, this indicates that specific attention should be paid to cervical screening from early middle age for users, or ex-users, of oral contraceptives.

Endometrial cancer

At least six studies (Weiss and Sayvetz, 1980; Kaufman et al., 1980; Hulka et al., 1982; La Vecchia et al., 1986; CASH, 1987a; World Health Organization, 1988) have found, with remarkable consistency in estimates, that oral contraceptive use is associated with significant protection against endometrial cancer. All the relative risks are close to their overall average of 0.5, indicating that oral contraceptive users, as a whole, have their risk of developing endometrial cancer reduced by about 50%. This protection increases with increasing duration of use, thus stressing the causal nature of the association, and appears to persist up to 10–15 years after stopping use. Since the continuous influence of oestrogenic substances unopposed by progesterone is at the present time firmly recognised as a major determinant of endometrial cancer (Kay and Pike, 1988), the protective effect of combined oral contraceptives was theoretically predictable. Endometrial mitotic activity, during which DNA copying errors are likely to occur, is virtually zero in women on combined oral contraceptives (Kay and Pike, 1988).

Endometrial cancer, nevertheless, is a rare disease in young and middle-aged women. Thus, in the absence of direct information about the possible persistence of the protection into older age, its proven impact should be considered, on a public health scale, as relatively limited.

Ovarian cancer

Epidemiological evidence about oral contraceptives and ovarian cancer is as clear and convincing as for endometrial cancer. Thirteen of 14 studies (Newhouse et al., 1977; Casagrande et al., 1979; Willett et al., 1981; Hildreth et al., 1981; Weiss et al., 1981; Cramer et al., 1982; Rosenberg et al., 1982; Tzonou et al., 1984; La Vecchia et al., 1986; CASH, 1987b; Harlow et al., 1988; Shu et al., 1989; World Health Organization, 1989; Booth et al., 1989) found RR below one. The overall estimate of protection of approximately 40% and a strong inverse relationship with duration of use have also been observed in most studies.

For ovarian cancer, too, protection has been shown to persist for some time (at least 10 years) after pill use has ceased. From a biological viewpoint, the beneficial effects of oral contraceptives on ovarian cancer risk have been interpreted chiefly in the framework of the 'incessant ovulation theory' (Casagrande et al., 1979). Ovariostasis, induced by oral contraceptives as well as by pregnancy and menopause, would avoid exposure of the ovarian epithelium to recurrent trauma and contact with follicular fluid.

Since the incidence of ovarian as opposed to endometrial cancer is already appreciable in middle age, and survival is substantially worse, the protection attributable to oral contraceptive use corresponds to avoidance of a far from negligible number of deaths (i.e. probably several hundreds per year in countries like Britain, where oral contraceptives have been used frequently for a long time).

Adenoma and cancer of the liver

It is known that oral contraceptives considerably increase (by at least a few dozen times) the risk of liver adenoma. There are few data about their impact on the risk of primary liver cancer, which may be due in some measure to the relative rarity of this disease.

Nevertheless, the five studies of the subject from developed countries (Henderson et al., 1983; Neuberger et al., 1986; Forman et al., 1986; La Vecchia et al., 1989; Palmer et al., 1989) found risks considerably above one for primary liver cancer in oral contraceptive users. The duration–risk relationship is very strong, with RR of the order of 10 for long-term use (over 5–8 years). However, primary liver cancer is extremely rare in younger women: therefore the absolute number of attributable cases is small, if not negligible. No case of primary liver cancer has been observed, for instance, in the cohort study of the Oxford Family Planning Association (Vessey et al., 1976), which included over 17 000 women followed for over two decades.

A multinational case–control study coordinated by the World Health Organization, chiefly conducted in developing countries and based on 36 histologically confirmed hepatocellular cancers, found no evidence of association (RR = 0.6) (World Health Organization, 1989). Although the frequency of long-term use was very low in that study, this may further indicate important differences in the determinants of hepatocellular carcinoma in various areas of the world.

Pituitary adenoma

Observation of upward trends in pituitary adenoma in Olmsted County, Minnesota (Annegers et al., 1978), led to the hypothesis of a direct relationship between oral contraceptives and the incidence of these tumours.

However, subsequent analyses of data from prospective (Wingrave et al., 1980) and case–control (Shy et al., 1983) studies did not support a causal nature of the association. In a study based on 72 incident cases from the State of Washington, for instance, the RR was 7.7 for women who used oral contraceptives for menstrual regulation, but only 1.3 (with 95% confidence interval of 0.7–2.6) for those who used the pill for birth control. This suggests that, in addition to impairment of diagnostic techniques for prolactinomas, the apparent association can be due to the use of oral contraceptives to treat menstrual irregularities of women with pituitary adenoma.

Cutaneous malignant melanoma

All the risk estimates in case–control studies (Beral et al., 1977; Adam et al., 1981; Bain et al., 1982; Holly et al., 1983; Helmrich et al., 1984; Beral et al., 1984; Holman et al., 1984; Gallagher et al., 1985; Green and Bain, 1985; Osterlind et al., 1988; Zanetti et al., 1990) except one (Beral et al., 1977) were close to one (between 0.7 and 1.2), providing evidence for the lack of any substantial association between oral contraceptives and cutaneous malignant melanoma. Thus, the summary RR was 0.9, with 95% confidence interval 0.7–1.0.

As in the retrospective investigations, no significant association between oral contraceptive use and cutaneous malignant melanoma risk emerged from a pooled analysis of three cohort studies (Vessey et al., 1976; Prentice and Thomas, 1987; Kay, 1981) and, most important, there was no trend of increasing risk with longer duration of use.

Conclusions

It is important to summarise some established concepts of the epidemiological evidence of adverse effects of oral contraceptives. First, epidemiological studies have produced important indications for intervention and prevention of vascular side-effects. Second, epidemiological evidence is clear, and remarkably consistent, in relation to female genital tract neoplasms (elevated risk for cervical, protection against endometrial and ovarian cancers), to the high RR for liver cancer in developed countries, and to the absence of a causal association for pituitary adenoma and skin melanoma. For breast cancer, overall evidence is consistent in showing elevated risks in women below age 35 who were long-term users, but no association in middle-aged women, at least with reference to currently available information. This leaves open major uncertainties in relation to the long-term effects of oral contraceptives on women's health (Vessey et al., 1989). It must be stated, however, that there is no indication that oral contraceptive use increases breast cancer risk among mature (>45 years old) women.

Breast cancer is, in fact, together with ovarian cancer, one of the key elements in any risk–benefit evaluation for middle-aged women (below age 50 or 55), while the public health impacts of all other diseases (including cardiovascular conditions) are comparably limited, if not negligible (Vessey et al., 1989).

ALTERNATIVE METHODS

Progestagen-only contraceptives

The progestin-only formulations contain no oestrogen. The tablets containing only progestin are taken daily, with no steroid-free interval.

This class of contraceptives relies heavily on progestational effects on cervical mucus, the endometrium, and tubal motility for effectiveness. The indications for using these agents are breast-feeding or inability to use oestrogen-containing agents. Unlike oestrogens, progestagens do not decrease the amount of lactation. No deleterious effect on the breast-feeding infant from the small amount of progestagen has been found (World Health Organization, 1984). Irregular bleeding occurs frequently with these agents, because no exogenous oestrogens are given, and the endogenous oestrogen levels are erratic due to the variable responses of the hypothalamic–pituitary axis. These bleeding irregularities are the most common reason for discontinuing the use of progestagen-only agents. Another problem with progestagen-only contraceptives is that they preferentially inhibit intrauterine pregnancy. When these agents fail, ectopic pregnancy must be carefully ruled out. The progestagen-only pill should be taken approximately the same time every evening. Its maximum effect on the cervical mucus is 3 h after oral ingestion, lasting approximately 18–24 h (Graham and Fraser, 1982).

The progestagen-only contraceptives delivered through depot preparations provide a more constant serum steroid level, avoiding the first-pass effect seen with oral administration. These delivery methods also have higher compliance rates, because a daily dose is not necessary (Diczfalusy, 1986). The first of these to be used was depo-medroxyprogesterone acetate. It is extremely effective and has been used worldwide for many years. The dosage is 150 mg every 3 months. Norethindrone enanthate is another injected progestagen, requiring an injection every 2 months. Both have similar efficacy, breakthrough bleeding rates, and termination rates of approximately 70% after 2 years (World Health Organization, 1983).

To extend the duration of action, progestagen implants have been developed. They provide reliable reversible contraception for 1–5 years. To have such a long duration, the potent progestagen, levonorgestral, is delivered from silastic-covered rods (Norplant) inserted subdermally or included in a biodegradable caproic acid form (Capronor).

Vaginal rings that constantly diffuse steroids from silastic tubing have been developed. The World Health Organization's Varlevo-20 is 55 mm in outer diameter and 9.5 mm in cross-sectional diameter. It is effective for 90 continuous days and contains levonorgestrel (Landgren et al., 1982). Male discomfort is reported to range from 8% to 24% (Faundes et al., 1981). Rings may be removed for up to 3 h for coitus and then reinserted without affecting the contraceptive effects.

Gonadotrophin-releasing hormone analogues

These compounds are currently given subcutaneously or intranasally. Depot formulations that have the advantage of avoiding daily administration have also been developed. When given continuously the GnRH analogues induce anovulation. In fact, if these compounds are given in a tonic fashion rather than a pulsatile fashion, there is an initial release of gonadotrophins, which leads to a decrease in gonadal steroid production. Therefore the possibility of using them as contraceptive agents was suggested (Thau, 1984; Nillus, 1985). In one study using the super-agonist, nafarelin acetate, given intranasally to 47 women in daily doses of 125–250 μg, anovulation was achieved in 261 of 262 treatment cycles (Gudmundsson et al., 1986). There were no pregnancies during the treatment period. Nine of the 47 women discontinued treatment because of vasomotor flushes. None of the women in the treatment group complained of dyspareunia or vaginal dryness. The treatment was readily reversible, with ovulatory cycles returning after a median time of 43 days following discontinuation of the GnRH agonist. The predominant uterine bleeding pattern was that of oligomenorrhoea, with bleeding occurring from 29 to 91 days, as average intervals. There is still concern about the long-term effects of this hypogonadotrophic state in terms of the risk of unopposed oestrogen and endometrial hyperplasia and of the metabolic effects on plasma lipids and possible acceleration of osteoporosis (Balmaceda et al., 1987).

GnRH agonists have been used for male subjects as well (Sundaram, 1984). They effectively decrease gonadotrophins and sperm counts, but also result in lowered testosterone, which is followed by a decrease in libido and impotence. Supplemental testosterone has been given with success. However, the long-term effects of this supplemental androgen require further investigation.

Antagonists of gonadotrophin-releasing hormone have also been developed. These agents competitively inhibit binding of GnRH to the receptor and can be displaced by GnRH. The clinical usefulness of these new drugs has yet to be determined.

Gossypol

Gossypol is a polyphenolic compound extracted from cottonseed oil. Gossypol appears to have several mechanisms of action, including inhibition of spermatogenesis, decreased sperm motility and function, and degeneration of seminiferous tubal epithelium. The compound is orally active and given as a loading dose followed by a lower maintenance dose (Liu et al., 1987).

Unfortunately the serious side-effects of Gossypol treatment, such as severe hypokalaemia and irreversible azoospermia, prevent its use by humans.

REFERENCES

Adam, S. A., Sheaves, J. K., Wright, N. H., Mosser, G. and Harris, R. W. (1981). A case–control study of the possible association between oral contraceptives and malignant melanoma. *Br. J. Cancer*, **44**, 45–50.

Adlercreutz, H., Martin, F., Jarventaa, T. and Fotsis, T. (1979). Steroid absorption and enterohepatic recycling. *Contraception*, **20**, 201–206.

Andolsek, L., Kovacic, U., Kozuh, M. and Litt, B. (1983). Oral contraceptives and cervical cancer. *Lancet*, **ii**, 1310–1315.

Annegers, J. F., Coulam, C. B. and Abbound, C. F. (1978). Pituitary adenoma in Olmsted County, Minnesota. *Mayo Clin. Proc.*, **53**, 641–643.

Back, B. J., Breckenridge, A. M., Crawford, E., Hall, J. M. and MacIver, M. (1980). The effect of rifampicin on the pharmacokinetics of ethinyl estradiol in women. *Contraception*, **21**, 135–141.

Bain, C., Hennekens, C. H., Speizer, F. E., Rosner, B. and Willett, W. (1982). Oral contraceptive use and malignant melanoma. *J. Natl. Cancer Inst.*, **68**, 537–539.

Balmaceda, J. P., Borrero, C. and Asch, R. H. (1987). Luteinising hormone-releasing hormone analogs: female contraception. *Semin. Reprod. Endocrinol.*, **5**, 371–372.

Beral, V., Ramcharan, S. and Faris, R. (1977). Malignant melanoma and oral contraceptive use among women in California. *Br. J. Cancer*, **36**, 804–809.

Beral, V., Evans, S. and Shaw, H. (1984). Oral contraceptive use and malignant melanoma in Australia. *Br. J. Cancer*, **50**, 681–685.

Booth, M., Beral, V. and Smith, P. (1989). Risk factors for ovarian cancer: a case–control study. *Br. J. Cancer*, **60**, 592–598.

Brenner, P. F., Mishell, D. R., Stanczyk, F. Z. and Goebelsmann, U. (1977). Serum levels of *d*-norgestrel, luteinizing hormone, follicle stimulating hormone, estradiol and progesterone in women during the following ingestion of oral contraceptives containing *dl*-norgestrel. *Am. J. Obstet. Gynecol.*, **129**, 133–138.

Brinton, L. A., Huggins, G. R., Lehman, H. F., Mallin, K. and Savitz, D. A. (1986). Long-term use of oral contraceptives and risk of invasive cervical cancer. *Int. J. Cancer*, **38**, 339–344.

Bruzzi, P., Negri, E., La Vecchia, C., Decarli, A. and Palli, D. (1988). Short term increase in risk of breast cancer after full term pregnancy. *Br. Med. J.*, **297**, 1096–1098.

Casagrande, J. T., Louie, E. W., Pike, M. C., Roy, S. and Ross, R. K. (1979). 'Incessant ovulation' and ovarian cancer. *Lancet*, **ii**, 170–172.

CASH: The Cancer and Steroid Hormone Study of the Centers for Disease Control and the National Institute of Child Health and Human Development (1987a). Combination oral contraceptive use and the risk of endometrial cancer. *JAMA*, **257**, 796–800.

CASH: The Cancer and Steroid Hormone Study of the Centers for Disease Control and the National Institute of Child Health and Human Development (1987b). The reduction in risk of ovarian cancer associated with oral-contraceptive use. *N. Engl. J. Med.*, **316**, 650–655.

Celentano, D. D., Klassen, A. C., Weisman, C. S. and Rosenshein, N. B. (1987). The role of contraceptive use in cervical cancer: the Maryland cervical cancer case–control study. *Am. J. Epidemiol.*, **126**, 592–604.

Chowdhury, V., Joshi, U. M., Gopalkrishna, K., Betrabet, S., Mehta, S. and Saxena, B. N. (1980). Escape ovulation in women due to the missing of low dose combination oral contraceptive pills. *Contraception*, **22**, 241–247.

Cramer, D. W., Hutchinson, G. B., Welch, W. R., Scully, R. E. and Kmapp, R. C. (1982). Factors affecting the association of oral contraceptives and ovarian cancer. *N. Engl. J. Med.*, **307**, 1047–1051.

De la Pena, A., Chenault, C. B. and Goldzieher, J. W. (1975). Radioimmunoassay of unconjugated plasma ethinylestradiol in women given a single oral dose of ethinyl estradiol as mestranol. *Steroids*, **25**, 773–776.

Delforge, J. P. and Ferin, J. (1970). The histometric study of 2 oestrogens: ethinyl oestradiol and its 3-methyl-ether derivative (mestranol): their comparative effect upon the growth of the human endometrium. *Contraception*, **1**, 57–62.

Diczfalusy, E. (1986). New developments in oral injectable and implantable contraceptives, vaginal rings and intrauterine devices: a review. *Contraception*, **33**, 7–12.

European Consensus Committee (1990). Consensus development meeting: metabolic aspects of oral contraceptives of relevance for cardiovascular diseases. *Am. J. Obstet. Gynecol.*, **162**, 1335–1337.

Fasal, E., Simmons, M. E. and Kampert, J. B. (1981). Factors associated with high and low risk of cervical neoplasia. *J. Natl. Cancer Inst.*, **66**, 631–636.

Faundes, A., Hardy, E., Reyes, C., Pastene, L. and Portes-Carrasco, R. (1981). Acceptability of the contraceptive vaginal ring by rural and urban populations in two Latin American countries. *Contraception*, **24**, 393–397.

Forman, D., Vincent, T. J. and Doll, R. (1986). Cancer of the liver and the use of oral contraceptives. *Br. Med. J.*, **292**, 1355–1359.

Gallagher, R. P., Elwood, J. M., Hill, G. B., Coldman, A. J. and Threlfall, W. J. (1985). Reproductive factors, oral contraceptives and risk of melanoma. Western Canada Melanoma Study. *Br. J. Cancer*, **52**, 901–907.

Grady, W. R., Hayward, M. D. and Yagi, J. (1986). Contraceptive failure in the United States: estimates from the 1982 National Survey of family growth. *Fam. Plann. Perspect.*, **18**, 200–203.

Graham, S. and Fraser, I. S. (1982). The progestogen-only mini-pill. *Contraception*, **26**, 373–377.

Green, A. and Bain, C. (1985). Hormonal factors and melanoma in women. *Med. J. Aust.*, **142**, 446–448.

Gudmundsson, J. A., Nillius, S. J. and Bergquist, C. (1986). Intranasal peptide contraception by inhibition of ovulation with gonadotrophin releasing hormone super agonist nafarelin: six months' clinical results. *Fertil. Steril.*, **45**, 817–821.

Harlow, B. L., Weiss, N. S., Roth, G. J., Chu, J. and Daling, J. R. (1988). Case–control study of borderline ovarian tumors: reproductive history and exposure to exogenous female hormones. *Cancer Res.*, **48**, 5849–5852.

Helmrich, S. P., Rosenberg, L., Kaufmann, D. W., Miller, D. R. and Schottenfeld, D. (1984). Lack of elevated risk of malignant melanoma in relation to oral contraceptive use. *J. Natl. Cancer Inst.*, **72**, 617–620.

Henderson, B. E., Preston-Martin, S., Edmondson, H. A., Peters, R. L. and Pike, M. C. (1983). Hepatocellular carcinoma and oral contraceptives. *Br. J. Cancer*, **48**, 437–441.

Hildreth, N. G., Kelsey, J. L., LiVolsi, V. A., Fischer, D. B. and Holford, T. R. (1981). An epidemiologic study of epithelial carcinoma of the ovary. *Am. J. Epidemiol.*, **114**, 398–405.

Holly, E. A., Weiss, N. S. and Liff, J. M. (1983). Cutaneous melanoma in relation to exogenous hormones and reproductive factors. *J. Natl. Cancer Inst.*, **70**, 827–831.

Holman, C. D. J., Armstrong, B. K. and Heenan, P. J. (1984). Cutaneous malignant melanoma in women: exogenous sex hormones and reproductive factors. *Br. J. Cancer*, **50**, 637–680.

Hulka, B. S., Chambless, L. E., Kaufmann, D. G., Fowler, W. C., Jr and Breenberg, B. G. (1982). Protection against endometrial carcinoma by combination-product oral contraceptives. *JAMA*, **247**, 475–477.

Irwin, K. L., Rosero-Bixby, L., Oberle, M. W., Lee, N. C. and Whatley, A. S. (1988). Oral contraceptives and cervical cancer risk in Costa Rica: detection bias or causal association? *JAMA*, **259**, 59–64.

Jick, H., Dinan, B. and Rothman, K. J. (1978). Oral contraceptives and nonfatal myocardial infarction. *JAMA*, **239**, 1403–1406.

Jick, S. S., Walker, A. M., Stergachis, A. and Jick, H. (1989). Oral contraceptives and breast cancer. *Br. J. Cancer*, **59**, 618–621.

Kappus, H. M. and Remmer, H. (1973). Affinity of ethinyl estradiol and mestranol for the uterine oestrogen receptor and for the microsomal mixed function oxidase of the liver. *J. Steroid Biochem.*, **4**, 121–124.

Kaufman, D. W., Shapiro, S., Slone, D., Rosenberg, L. and Miettinen, O. S. (1980). Decreased risk of endometrial cancer among oral-contraceptive users. *N. Engl. J. Med.*, **303**, 1045–1047.

Kay, C. R. (1981). Malignant melanoma and oral contraceptives. *Br. J. Cancer*, **44**, 479–482.

Kay, C. R. and Hannaford, P. C. (1988). Breast cancer and the pill: a further report from the Royal College of General Practitioners' oral contraception study. *Br. J. Cancer*, **58**, 675–680.

Kay, T. J. A. and Pike, M. C. (1988). The dose–effect relationship between 'unopposed' oestrogens and endometrial mitotic rate: its central role in explaining and predicting endometrial cancer risk. *Br. J. Cancer*, **57**, 205–212.

Landgren, B. M., Johannison, E., Masironi, B. and Dicafalnsy, E. (1982). Pharmacokinetic and pharmacodynamic investigations with vaginal devices releasing levonorgestrel at a constant, near zero rate. *Contraception*, **26**, 567–572.

Larrea, F., Vilchis, F., Chavez, B., Perez, A., Garza-Flores, J. and Perez-Palacios, G. (1987). The metabolism of 19-nor contraceptive progestins modulates the biological activity at the neuroendocrine level. *J. Steroid Biochem.*, **27**, 657–661.

La Vecchia, C., Decarli, A., Fasoli, M., Franceschi, S. and Gentile A. (1986). Oral contraceptives and cancers of the breast and of the female genital tract: interim results from a case–control study. *Br. J. Cancer*, **54**, 311–317.

La Vecchia, C., Negri, E. and Parazzini, F. (1989). Oral contraceptives and primary liver cancer. *Br. J. Cancer*, **59**, 460–461.

Liu, G. Z., Lyle, K. C. and Cao, J. (1987). Experiences with gossypol as a male pill. *Am. J. Obstet. Gynecol.*, **157**, 1079–1081.

Lubin, J. H., Burns, P. E., Blot, W. J., Lees, A. W. and May, C. (1982). Risk factors for breast cancer in women in Northern Alberta, Canada, as related to age at diagnosis. *J. Natl. Cancer Inst.*, **68**, 211–217.

Mann, J. I., Inman, W. H. W. and Thorogood, M. (1976). Oral contraceptive use in older women and fatal myocardial infarction. *Br. Med. J.*, **2**, 445–447.

McPherson, K., Coope, P. A. and Vessey, M. P. (1986). Early oral contraceptive use and breast cancer: theoretical effects of latency. *J. Epidemiol. Community Health*, **40**, 289–294.

McPherson, K., Vessey, M. P., Neil, A., Doll, R. and Jones, L. (1987). Early oral contraceptive use and breast cancer: results of another case–control study. *Br. J. Cancer*, **56**, 653–660.

Meirik, O., Lund, E., Adami, H. O., Bergström, R. and Christoffersen, T. (1986). Oral contraceptive use and breast cancer in young women: a joint national case–control study in Sweden and Norway. *Lancet*, **ii**, 650–654.

Miale, J. B. and Kent, J. W. (1974). The effects of oral contraceptives on results of laboratory tests. *Am. J. Obstet. Gynecol.*, **120**, 264–269.

Miller, D. R., Rosenberg, L., Kaufman, D. W., Stolley, P. and Warshauer, M. E. (1989). Breast cancer before age 45 and oral contraceptive use: new findings. *Am. J. Epidemiol.*, **129**, 269–280.

Molina, R., Thomas, D. B., Dabancens, A., Lopez, J. and Ray, R. M. (1988). Oral contraceptives and cervical carcinoma in situ in Chile. *Cancer Res.*, **48**, 1011–1015.

Morris, S. E., Groom, G. V., Cameron, E. D., Buckingham, M. S., Everitt, J. M. and Elstein, M. (1979). Studies on low dose oral contraceptives: plasma hormone changes in relation to deliberate pill (microgynon 30) omission. *Contraception*, **20**, 61–68.

Murphy, M. F. G., Campbell, M. J. and Bone, M. (1989). Is there an increased risk of twinning after discontinuation of the oral contraceptive pill? *J. Epidemiol. Community Health*, **43**, 275–279.

Neuberger, J., Forman, D., Doll, R. and Williams, R. (1986). Oral contraceptives and hepatocellular carcinoma. *Br. Med. J.*, **292**, 1355–1361.

Newhouse, M. L., Pearson, R. M., Fullerton, J. M., Boesen, E. A. M. and Shannon, H. S. (1977). A case–control study of carcinoma of the ovary. *Br. J. Prevent. Social Med.*, **31**, 148–155.

Nillus, S. J. (1985). Gonadotrophin releasing hormone analogs for female contraception by inhibition of ovulation. *J. Steroid Biochem.*, **23**, 849–855.

Olsson, H., Möller, T. R. and Ranstam, J. (1989). Early oral contraceptive use and breast cancer among premenopausal women: final report from a study in Southern Sweden. *J. Natl. Cancer Inst.*, **81**, 1000–1004.

Ory, H. W., Conger, S. B., Naib, Z., Tyler, C. W. Jr and Hatcher, R. A. (1977). Preliminary analysis of oral contraceptive use and risk of developing premalignant lesion of the uterine cervix. In S. Garattini and Berendes (eds), *Pharmacology of Steroid Contraceptive Drugs*. Raven Press, New York, pp. 211–224.

Osterlind, A., Tucker, M. A., Stone, B. J. and Jensen, O. M. (1988). The Danish case–control study of cutaneous malignant melanoma. III. Hormonal and reproductive factors in women. *Int. J. Cancer*, **42**, 821–824.

Palmer, J. R., Rosenberg, L., Kaufman, D. W., Warshauer, M. E. and Stolley P. (1989). Oral contraceptive use and liver cancer. *Am. J. Epidemiol.*, **130**, 878–882.

Paul, Ch., Skegg, D. C. G., Spears, G. F. S. and Kaldor, J. M. (1986). Oral contraceptives and breast cancer: a national study. *Br. Med. J.*, **293**, 723–726.

Pike, M. C., Henderson, B. E., Krailo, M. D., Duke, A. and Roy, S. (1983). Breast cancer in young women and use of oral contraceptives: possible modifying effect of formulation and age at use. *Lancet*, **ii**, 926–930.

Prentice, R. L. and Thomas, D. B. (1987). On the epidemiology of oral contraceptives and disease. *Adv. Cancer Res.*, **49**, 285–401.

Ramcharan, S., Pellegrin, F. A., Ray, R. and Hsu, J. P. (1981). A prospective study of the side effects of oral contraceptives. *The Walnut Creek Contraceptive Study* (Vol. III). NIH Publication No. 81–564, Bethesda, MD.

Ravnihar, B., Zakelj, M. P., Kosmelj, K. and Stare, J. (1988). A case–control study of breast cancer in relation to oral contraceptive use in Slovenia. *Neoplasma*, **35**, 109–121.

Reed, M. J., Fortherby, K., Steel, S. J. and Addison, J. (1972). In vivo and in vitro metabolism of ethinyl estradiol. *J. Endocrinol.*, **53**, 28–33.

Romieu, I., Willett, W. C., Colditz, G. A., Stampfer, M. J. and Rosner, B. (1989). Prospective study of oral contraceptive use and risk of breast cancer in women. *J. Natl. Cancer Inst.*, **81**, 1313–1321.

Rosenberg, L., Shapiro, S., Slone, D., Kaufman, D. W. and Helmrich, S. P. (1982). Epithelial ovarian cancer and combination oral contraceptives. *JAMA*, **247**, 3210–3212.

Rosenberg, L., Miller, D. R., Kaufman, D. W., Helmrich, S. P. and Stolley, P. D. (1984). Breast cancer and oral contraceptive use. *Am. J. Epidemiol.*, **119**, 167–176.

Rosenberg, L., Palmer, J. R., Lesko, S. M. and Shapiro, S. (1990). Oral contraceptives and the risk of myocardial infarction. *Am. J. Epidemiol.*, **131**, 1009–1016.

Royal College of General Practitioners (1974). Oral contraceptives and health: an interim report from the Oral Contraception Study of the Royal College of General Practitioners. Pitman Medical, London.

Shapiro, S., Slone, D., Rosenberg, L., Kaufman, D. W. and Stolley, P. D. (1979). Oral-contraceptive use in relation to myocardial infarction. *Lancet*, **i**, 743–747.

Shu, X. O., Brinton, L. A., Gao, Y. T. and Yuan, J. M. (1989). Population-based case–control study of ovarian cancer in Shanghai. *Cancer Res.*, **49**, 3670–3674.

Shy, K. K., McTiernan, A. M., Daling, J. R. and Weiss, N. S. (1983). Oral contraceptive use and the occurrence of pituitary prolactinoma. *JAMA*, **249**, 2204–2207.

Stadel, B. V. (1981). Oral contraceptives and cardiovascular disease. *N. Engl. J. Med.*, **305**, 612–618.

Stadel, B. V., Rubin, G. L., Webster, L. A., Schlesselman, J. J. and Wingo, P. A. (1985). Oral contraceptives and breast cancer in young women. *Lancet*, **ii**, 970–973.

Stampfer, M. J., Willett, W. C., Colditz, G. A., Speizer, F. E. and Hennekens, C. H. (1988). A prospective study of past use of oral contraceptive agents and risk of cardiovascular diseases. *N. Engl. J. Med.*, **319**, 1313–1317.

Stanford, J. L., Brinton, L. A. and Hoover, R. N. (1989). Oral contraceptives and breast cancer: results from an expanded case–control study. *Br. J. Cancer*, **60**, 375–381.

Sundaram, K. (1984). Use of LHRH agonists and antagonists in male contraception: A review. *Contraception*, **29**, 163–171.

Thau, R. B. (1984). Luteinising hormone releasing hormone (LHRH) and its analogs for contraception in women: a review. *Contraception*, **29**, 143–149.

The WHO Collaborative Study of Neoplasia and Steroid Contraceptives (1989). *Int. J. Cancer*, **43**, 254–259.

Thomas, D. B. (1972). Relationship of oral contraceptives to cervical carcinogenesis. *Obstet. Gynecol.*, **40**, 508–518.

Tzonou, A., Day, N. E., Trichopoulos, D., Walker, A. and Saliaraki, M. (1984). The epidemiology of ovarian cancer in Greece: a case–control study. *Eur. J. Cancer Clin. Oncol.*, **20**, 1045–1052.

Vessey, M. P. and Doll, R. (1968). Investigation of relation between use of oral contraceptives and thromboembolic disease. *Br. Med. J.*, **ii**, 199–205.

Vessey, M., Doll, R., Peto, R., Johnson, B. and Wiggins, P. (1976). A long-term follow-up study of women using different methods of contraception: an interim report. *J. Biosoc. Sci.*, **8**, 373–427.

Vessey, M. P., Villard-Mackintosh, L., McPherson, K. and Yeates, D. (1989). Mortality among oral contraceptive users: 20 year follow up of women in a cohort study. *Br. Med. J.*, **299**, 1487–1491.

Wah, R. and Barbieri, R. (1988). Hormonal contraceptive agents. In *Reproductive Endocrine Therapeutics*, A. R. Liss Inc., New York, pp. 351–389.

Weiss, N. S. and Sayvetz, T. A. (1980). Incidence of endometrial cancer in relation to the use of oral contraceptives. *N. Engl. J. Med.*, **302**, 551–554.

Weiss, N. S., Lyon, J. L., Liff, J. M., Vollmer, W. M. and Daling, J. R. (1981). Incidence of ovarian cancer in relation to the use of oral contraceptives. *Int. J. Cancer*, **28**, 669–671.

World Health Organization (1983). Multinational comparative clinical evaluations of long acting injectable contraceptive steroids: norethisterone enanthate and depot medroxyprogesterone acetate. Final report. *Contraception*, **28**, 1–9.

World Health Organization: Task force on oral contraceptives (1984). Effects of hormonal contraceptives on milk volume and infant growth. *Contraception*, **30**, 505–514.

WHO Collaborative Study of Neoplasia and Steroid Contraceptives (1985). Invasive cervical cancer and combined oral contraceptives. *Br. Med. J.*, **290**, 961–965.

WHO Collaborative Study of Neoplasia and Steroid Contraceptives (1988). Endometrial cancer and combined oral contraceptives. *Int. J. Epidemiol.*, **17**, 263–269.

WHO Collaborative Study of Neoplasia and Steroid Contraceptives (1989). Epithelial ovarian cancer and combined oral contraceptives. *Int. J. Epidemiol.*, **18**, 538–545.

Willett, W. C., Bain, C., Hennekens, C. H., Rosner, B. and Speizer, F. E. (1981). Oral contraceptives and risk of ovarian cancer. *Cancer*, **48**, 1684–1687.

Wilson, J. G. and Brent, R. L. (1981) Are female hormones teratogenic? *Am. J. Obstet. Gynecol.*, **141**, 567–572.

Wingrave, S. J., Kay, C. R. and Vessey, M. P. (1980). Oral contraceptives and pituitary adenomas. *Br. Med. J.*, **i**, 686–698.

Zanetti, R., Franceschi, S., Rosso, S., Bidoli, E. and Colonna, S. (1990). Cutaneous malignant melanoma in females: the role of hormonal and reproductive factors. *Int. J. Epidemiol.*, **19**, 522–526.

10

The Menopause

Adam Rodin and Michael Chapman
Guy's Hospital, London, UK

The menopause is defined as the ending of menstruation and it marks the end of a woman's reproductive potential. Ovarian failure, which underlies the menopause, results in oestrogen deficiency, and this is responsible for the short-term and long-term sequelae of the menopause.

During the twentieth century both the reproductive and total lifespans of women have increased gradually. The prolongation of the reproductive era is primarily due to the earlier appearance of the menarche. The age of the menopause has not changed since medieval times and before the end of the nineteenth century fewer than 30% of women reached the menopause. With improved life expectancy the post-menopausal years have achieved greater importance. The average age of the menopause in the UK is 51 years and as average female life expectancy is over 80 years, women may spend up to 40% of their lives after the menopause.

Little is known about the factors which determine age at menopause. It does not appear to be related to age of menarche, socio-economic factors, race, parity, weight or height. Cigarette smoking may predispose to earlier menopause. The menopause may be 'iatrogenic' and may follow surgical procedures, most commonly bilateral oophorectomy or irradiation. There is evidence that women who undergo total abdominal hysterectomy with conservation of ovaries subsequently undergo earlier ovarian failure and this may be due to compromised ovarian blood supply. About 8% of women undergo a premature menopause (<40 years). This may be due to autoimmune disease and may rarely be associated with myasthenia gravis, idiopathic thrombocytopenic purpura, rheumatoid arthritis, vitiligo and autoimmune haemolytic anaemia.

Understanding Common Disorders in Reproductive Endocrinology. Edited by M.M. Dooley and M.P. Brincat.

The term 'La Menespausie' was first used in 1861 when De Gardanne recognized the syndrome of complaints associated with the ending of menstruation. Since then it has been established that the numerous manifestations of the menopause syndrome are due to oestrogen deficiency and that these can be successfully managed with oestrogen replacement therapy.

ENDOCRINOLOGY OF THE CLIMACTERIC AND THE MENOPAUSE

In pre-menopausal women the main oestrogen is 17β-oestradiol, which is synthesised by the granulosa cells of the developing ovarian follicles. In the normal non-pregnant female oestradiol is produced at an average rate of 100–300 μg per day; however, this varies widely during the ovarian cycle. In addition, oestrogen is also produced by the peripheral conversion of androstenedione to oestrone. Androstenedione is secreted by the ovaries and the adrenal glands and is converted to oestrone in adipose tissue by aromatisation. The rate of extraglandular oestrone formation does not vary significantly during the cycle.

The climacteric is the transition phase that precedes the menopause and it may last 10–15 years. It is characterised by reduced sensitivity of the remaining ovarian follicles to stimulation by gonadotrophins. As a result, ovulation becomes less frequent, total monthly oestrogen production declines and peak gonadotrophin levels may be elevated. It is not uncommon for women to experience symptoms of oestrogen deficiency during the climacteric. Menstruation may remain regular; however, erratic cycles and menorrhagia are characteristic features of the climacteric and are due to anovulation and failure of corpus luteum formation.

At the menopause, the ovaries fail to respond to the gonadotrophins and oestrogen production is insufficient to cause the endometrium to proliferate, resulting in the cessation of menstruation. There is a 10- to 20-fold increase in follicle-stimulating hormone (FSH) and a three-fold increase in luteinising hormone (LH), reaching a peak 2 years after the menopause and then gradually declining. After the menopause oestrogen production by the ovaries ceases and oestrone is the main circulating oestrogen. This is a weaker oestrogen than 17β-oestradiol and is produced from androstenedione in adipose tissue and a variety of other sites, including skin, hair follicles, brain, bone and muscle. Androstenedione is derived mainly from the adrenal gland, with a small amount secreted by the ovarian stroma. The average production rate of oestrogen in the post-menopausal woman is approximately 45 μg per 24 h. Conversion of androstenedione correlates with body weight, which correlates positively with circulating levels of oestrone, and this explains the well-recognised association between obesity and endometrial carcinoma.

Testosterone secretion by the post-menopausal ovary continues under the influence of elevated gonadotrophin levels which stimulates the ovarian stroma. Oestrogen derived from extraglandular sources may be sufficient to sustain oestrogen-sensitive tissues initially but with increasing age this proves inadequate and atrophy occurs.

THE MENOPAUSE SYNDROME

The effects of oestrogen deficiency are many and varied, and it is only in recent years that the full spectrum of sequelae has been recognised. Oestrogen deficiency results in short-term and long-term effects, and individuals vary in the pattern and severity of complications that they suffer. Approximately 75% of women experience symptoms at the time of the menopause. Those who avoid the short-term problems are not protected from the important late effects of oestrogen lack. The short-term consequences of the menopause can be conveniently considered in two categories: physical and psychological effects (Table 1).

Symptoms of vasomotor instability and psychological problems tend to predominate in the climacteric and in the early post-menopausal era, while complications due to end organ atrophy are most common in the later post-menopausal years.

Vasomotor instability

Hot flushes and night sweats are the most widely recognised manifestations of the menopause. They affect 75–85% of women experiencing a natural menopause or who undergo bilateral oophorectomy, and in 25% of cases they are severely disruptive. They usually persist for over 12 months and in 25% of women they continue for more than 5 years. Flushes commonly occur during the climacteric. They may be precipitated by a variety of everyday activities but most commonly there is no identifiable trigger. Women describe a sudden sensation of heat in the face and neck that spreads to the

Table 1 The short-term consequences of oestrogen deficiency

Physical	Psychological
Vasomotor instability	Depression/anxiety
End organ atrophy	Irritability
Genital tract	Poor memory/concentration
Other sites	Sexual dysfunction
Lethargy/fatigue	

chest. This usually lasts for several minutes and is often accompanied by a visible red flush and perspiration, which may be profuse. During these episodes women may experience palpitations, nausea and dizziness. Hot flushes occurring during sleep are known as night sweats and result in sleep deprivation.

During a flush the finger temperature characteristically rises by 7.5 °F and then returns to normal in about 30 min. Core temperature falls during a flush and it is proposed that the hot flush is triggered by a sudden downward resetting of the central thermoregulatory centre. The aetiology of vasomotor instability is uncertain although it is initiated by the withdrawal of oestrogen. Flushes are accompanied by a pulse of LH secretion from the pituitary, but this is not causative. It is likely that flushes are determined by events in the hypothalamus, and the role of catecholamines and β-endorphins is under investigation.

End organ atrophy

Deficiency of oestrogen leads to progressive atrophy of tissues at various sites. The tissues most severely affected are those that carry the highest concentrations of oestrogen receptors, in particular the urogenital tract and the breasts.

The vulva undergoes atrophy, with a reduction in size of the labia majora and loss of pubic hair. The vaginal epithelium is highly responsive to oestrogen. After the menopause the vagina becomes slightly shortened and thinned and histologically there is loss of glycogen and flattening of the epithelium. Vaginal atrophy leads to vaginal dryness and dyspareunia. In addition, a thin-walled vagina is vulnerable to mechanical injury and readily bleeds. Atrophic vaginitis is a common cause of post-menopausal bleeding. After the menopause vaginal pH rises above 5 owing to the loss of lactic acid-producing Doderlein's bacilli, which are glycogen-dependent. This results in changes in the vaginal microflora and an increased risk of infections.

The cervix often becomes flush with the vaginal vault, and the squamocolumnar junction retreats into the endocervical canal. The uterine body reduces in size and the endometrium becomes atrophic, with a flattened non-proliferating epithelium and glands lined by only a single layer of cells. Laxity developing in the 'ligaments' that support the genital tract may result in the appearance of prolapse after the menopause.

Lower urinary tract dysfunction is common in women after the menopause; however, it is unclear whether this is a consequence of oestrogen deficiency following ovarian failure or whether this is age-related. The distal urethra is affected by similar atrophic changes to those of the vagina, and the transitional epithelium of the bladder responds to oestrogen like the vaginal epithelium. Frequency, urgency and urge incontinence appear to respond well to oestrogen replacement but there is little evidence that stress incontinence is improved.

During the post-menopausal years the breasts become atrophic, with a reduction in the amount of adipose tissue and lobules and replacement by fibrous tissue. The skin and its appendages are also maintained by oestrogen. After the menopause, skin collagen content falls and skin becomes thin, with a loss of elasticity. Arthralgia may be due to laxity in the support structures around joints and often responds well to oestrogen replacement therapy.

Psychological symptoms

Psychological symptoms are common in women of menopausal age, and studies have shown an incidence of psychological pathology of over 80% among attenders of menopause clinics. These symptoms often predate the ending of menstruation and are common during the climacteric. Depression and anxiety are frequent complaints, but loss of memory and confidence and poor concentration are particularly distressing. Debate continues about the aetiology of the psychological problems associated with the menopause. Some argue that there is a direct effect of oestrogen deficiency and they cite the finding of oestrogen receptors in the central nervous system as evidence for this. Others have demonstrated that there is a clustering of stressful life events in women in this age group, and total life stresses appear to peak at about the same time as psychological symptoms. It has also been suggested that psychological symptoms are secondary to disruptive physical problems and that a 'domino effect' operates. It seems likely that all three mechanisms contribute to the excess of psychological difficulties experienced by women in this age group.

THE LONG-TERM CONSEQUENCES OF THE MENOPAUSE

The long-term consequences of oestrogen deficiency following the menopause are osteoporosis and cardiovascular disease. Both of these conditions are 'silent' in their early stages but are important causes of morbidity and mortality in the ageing female population.

Osteoporosis

Osteoporosis is defined as a reduction in the mass of bone per unit volume throughout the skeleton, leading to fracture following minimal trauma. There are various causes of osteoporosis, but post-menopausal osteoporosis is the commonest form. Albright was the first to recognise the importance of oestrogen for the maintenance of skeletal integrity 50 years ago.

The development of osteoporosis in an individual depends on the peak adult bone mass achieved and the subsequent rate of bone loss. Peak bone mass is reached in the mid-thirties and it appears to be largely determined by genetic factors, although environmental determinants such as diet and exercise may contribute. At skeletal maturity men have 30–50% higher bone mass than women. Bone loss commences during the climacteric and continues at a slow rate until the menopause. Following the menopause, oestrogen deficiency results in a period of accelerated bone loss which continues for approximately 5 years. During this time bone loss proceeds exponentially at a rate of 2–5% per year and subsequently levels off. The majority of this loss is from the trabecular component of bone. A lower peak bone mass and the accelerated period of bone loss after the menopause explains why osteoporosis is commoner in women. The mechanism by which oestrogen protects the skeleton remains obscure. Its primary action is the inhibition of bone resorption, and in the past it was thought to act indirectly via the calcitrophic hormones, vitamin D, parathyroid hormone and calcitonin. In 1988, oestradiol receptors were identified on osteoblasts, providing a mechanism by which oestrogen might act directly.

Although other factors such as frequency of falls are important, the amount of bone present is the single most important factor determining the likelihood of fracture. A variety of non-invasive techniques have been developed that allow precise and accurate measurement of bone density at the clinically important sites where fractures tend to occur (vertebral bodies, neck of femur, distal radius). Those methods in current use include quantitative computed tomography and photon absorptiometry. The most recent advance in absorptiometry has been the introduction of dual-energy X-ray absorptiometry. In this technique, an X-ray source is used and dual energies are obtained by either switching kilovoltage or by filtering X-rays from a stable X-ray tube. A highly collimated X-ray beam is directed at the measurement site and the transmitted beam intensity is recorded via a detector. The region of interest is scanned and a point-by-point determination of bone mineral is made. This technique is rapid and radiation exposure is low.

In the presence of osteoporosis, fracture of any bone can occur, but the most common fractures are of the hip, vertebral bodies and distal radius (Colles' fracture). Hip fractures are commoner in women than men (2:1) and their incidence increases exponentially with age. In 1985 the number of hip fractures in England and Wales was 46 000 and the age-specific incidence is increasing for unknown reasons. Hip fracture is associated with significant morbidity and mortality. Up to 25% of affected individuals die as a result of the fracture or complications that follow, and only a minority of patients regain their former mobility. Vertebral fractures are common and by the age of 70 years it is estimated that 25% of women will have suffered at least one vertebral fracture. They may be painless and progressive, presenting with height loss and deformity, or they may be acute, accompanied by severe back pain. The incidence of Colles' fracture increases among women after the menopause but then reaches a plateau, unlike vertebral or hip fractures. Treatment of established osteoporosis is difficult and unrewarding, and efforts are now turning towards prophylaxis (see Benefits of hormone replacement therapy, below).

Cardiovascular disease

Cardiovascular disease is the leading cause of death in the developed world. Between the ages of 35 and 44 years coronary heart disease (CHD) mortality is approximately six times higher in men than women. However, by the age of 50 years mortality in men is only twofold higher and by the age of 70 years male and female rates of cardiovascular disease are indistinguishable. Loss of ovarian activity appears to result in an increased risk of cardiovascular disease. This is supported by the observation that women who have undergone a premature menopause have a higher risk of atherosclerosis and CHD mortality. Oestrogen has been identified as the likely factor that protects pre-menopausal women from CHD. The mechanism of this protective effect is still under investigation but it seems that a substantial benefit is obtained through its influence on the plasma lipid profile.

The major lipids found in human plasma are triglycerides, phospholipids and cholesterol esters. These molecules are all esters of long-chain fatty acids and together they comprise the lipid part of lipoproteins. Free fatty acids are also found in plasma.

Triglycerides are fatty acid esters of glycerol, which may be synthesised in the small intestine, liver or adipose tissue. Dietary triglycerides are absorbed in the form of chylomicrons, which reach the systemic circulation via the thoracic duct. Triglycerides made from endogenous fatty acids are mainly formed in the liver and they are secreted in the form of very-low-density lipoproteins (VLDL). Triglycerides have a relatively short half-life in plasma and are mainly removed by adipose tissue. Chylomicron triglyceride should have been removed within 12 h of a fatty meal, and measurement of plasma levels in the fasting state reflects the amount of endogenous triglyceride in the circulation.

Phospholipids and cholesterol are integral parts of all cell membranes and they exist in the plasma as constituents of lipoproteins. All lipids are transported in the plasma in the form of lipoproteins. These complex structures comprise an outer shell made up of phospholipids, cholesterol and apoproteins surrounding a core containing triglycerides and cholesterol esters. Ultracentrifugation of post-prandial plasma yields six distinct classes of lipoprotein which differ in size and composition (Table 2).

Table 2 The lipoproteins

	Mean diameter (nm)	% Protein	% Lipid
Chylomicron	100–1000	2	98
VLDL	43	10	90
IDL	27	18	82
LDL	22	25	75
HDL2	10	40	60
HDL3	7	55	45

Low-density lipoprotein (LDL) is the main cholesterol-carrying particle in the plasma and is derived from VLDL. It contains apoprotein B. High-density lipoprotein (HDL) contains apoproteins A–1 and A–2. HDL is subdivided into HDL2 and HDL3. Epidemiological studies have demonstrated that risk of CHD is correlated with concentrations of certain lipids and lipoproteins. Rising levels of total cholesterol, LDL, apoprotein B and probably triglycerides are associated with an increasing incidence of CHD, and it is suggested that LDL plays a direct role in the pathogenesis of atheroma. There is an inverse correlation between HDL and CHD risk but the mechanism by which HDL protects against CHD is yet to be established.

Plasma lipid and lipoprotein levels are influenced by age, sex and genetic factors, as well as by diet, smoking, body weight and physical activity. Women tend to have lower triglyceride and VLDL levels and higher HDL2 levels than men from puberty onwards. Their total and LDL cholesterol levels are lower until the menopause but afterwards become higher than in men of a similar age.

The favourable lipid profile in pre-menopausal women is maintained by the influence of oestrogen, which tends to elevate HDL and suppress LDL levels. After the menopause, this beneficial profile can be regained by the use of oestrogen replacement therapy. The addition of progestagens (see below) may counteract the cardioprotective effect of oestrogen on the lipid profile by suppressing HDL and elevating LDL. Progestagens vary in their effects on lipids/lipoproteins, and the more androgenic compounds have the greatest negative influence. There are concerns that the addition of progestagens to hormone replacement regimes may diminish the oestrogen-induced protection from CHD (see Benefits of hormone replacement therapy, below).

It is currently estimated that approximately 30% of the cardioprotective effect of oestrogen is derived from its influence of the lipid profile. Oestrogens may affect the prostaglandin/thromboxane system, causing vascular dilatation and reduced platelet aggregation, and it seems likely that cardioprotection may be achieved by a variety of mechanisms.

MANAGEMENT OF THE CLIMACTERIC AND POST-MENOPAUSAL YEARS

The introduction of hormone replacement therapy (HRT) over 25 years ago followed the recognition that the diverse problems seen in women in the climacteric and post-menopausal years are due to oestrogen deficiency and should be treated by appropriate supplementation.

The oestrogens used in current HRT preparations are natural and this distinguishes them from the synthetic oestrogens used in the combined oral contraceptive pill. Unlike the potent oestrogens used in the pill, they do significantly influence coagulation, fibrinolysis or carbohydrate metabolism. The natural oestrogens which are in common use in HRT preparations are conjugated equine oestrogens derived from the urine of pregnant mares, oestradiol valerate and 17β-oestradiol. When HRT was first introduced oestrogens alone were prescribed for 21 days each month. By the mid-1970s it became apparent that women treated with unopposed oestrogen were at risk of irregular vaginal bleeding, endometrial hyperplasia and carcinoma of the endometrium. The incidence of carcinoma of the endometrium was one in 1000 women per annum in untreated women, and this increased to four per 1000 women per annum in oestrogen-treated women. Although the tumours that developed in these women were usually well differentiated and prognosis was excellent, the increased risk of carcinoma of the endometrium was cumulative with each year of oestrogen use. Concerns about the increased incidence of endometrial cancer led to the addition of cyclical progestagen therapy to oestrogen replacement regimens. An adequate dose of progestagen taken for 12–14 days each not only eliminates the increased relative risk but reduces the incidence of endometrial cancer in treated patients to below that of the untreated population.

The addition of a progestagen may have unwanted effects, and up to 20% of HRT users discontinue treatment owing to progestagen-related side-effects. Foremost among these is the resumption of menstruation, which occurs in over 80% of women with an intact uterus. In addition, some women experience troublesome pre-menstrual symptoms while taking progestagen. The effects of progestagen on lipids has been discussed previously. There has been some interest in the use of continuous low-dose progestagen used with continuous oestrogen replacement. This regime successfully produces amenorrhoea in some women although a significant proportion will experience irregular bleeding.

TREATMENT REGIMES OF HORMONE REPLACEMENT THERAPY

Treatment may be tailored to suit individual requirements by altering oestrogen dose and route of administration. In addition, progestagen type and dose may be varied and it may be given cyclically or continuously. In general, oestrogen should be given continuously and at a constant dosage. Following hysterectomy, women should receive continuous unopposed oestrogen replacement. The addition of a progestagen is unnecessary as endometrial protection is no longer a concern.

Choice of oestrogen

Oral administration of oestrogen has the benefit of well-documented positive side-effects on the lipid profile and prevention of osteoporosis. Parenteral (transdermal or subcutaneous) administration of oestrogen avoids the liver first-pass effect and delivers the hormones directly into the bloodstream.

The major side-effect of transdermal therapy is skin irritation, which occurs in up to 20% of patients. Application to the buttocks with regular site rotation helps reduce the incidence of skin irritation. Subcutaneous implants improve patient compliance and have been reported to deliver physiological levels and physiological oestradiol to oestriol levels. With implants compliance is good but the problem of tachyphylaxis can occur. The different oestrogens available can be seen in Table 3.

Choice of progestin

Since progestins may have an adverse effect on cardiovascular risk the lowest dose needed to prevent endometrial hyperplasia should be used.

The minimum effective daily dose of various orally administered progestagens when added for 10–12 days of each calendar month are:

Norethisterone 0.7–2.5 mg
L-Norgestrel 150 mg
Dydrogestrone 10–20 mg
Medroxyprogesterone acetate 10 mg

Continuous therapy to give endometrial atrophy includes doses of 2.5 mg of medroxyprogesterone acetate daily or 0.35 mg norethisterone acetate.

Tibolone, a synthetic steroid, has progestagenic, androgenic and

Table 3 Oestrogens available for hormone replacement

	Daily dose
Conjugated equine oestrogens	0.625–1.25 mg
Oestradiol valerate	1–2 mg
Transdermal oestradiol	25–100 μg
Oestradiol implant	25–100 mg

oestrogenic effects, and continuous administration provides short-term and possibly long-term benefits without vaginal bleeding.

Transdermal progestins are available in a cyclic regime and hyperplastic endometrium is avoided.

Indications for considering HRT in an individual are listed in Table 4. A detailed history is taken when a woman first attends clinic. The presenting symptoms are recorded and an assessment is made of their severity. Some symptoms are embarrassing or distressing and may not be volunteered without direct questioning. A gynaecological history is taken and, in particular, the patient is asked about abnormal bleeding patterns or the occurrence of post-menopausal bleeding. Obstetric history is noted and a detailed general medical history is elicited. Current medication is also noted although adverse drug interactions are rare with HRT. A family history of osteoporosis or heart disease may have prompted attendance, and a family history of carcinoma of the breast may cause concerns about commencing HRT. Details of social circumstances should also be taken. Contraindications to HRT should be excluded (Table 5). Carcinoma of the breast and endometrium are oestrogen-dependent tumours. HRT is avoided in women with a history of either malignancy as there is concern about promoting recurrent disease.

A general physical examination is performed, and height and weight are recorded. Pelvic examination is carried out to exclude pelvic masses, and a cervical smear is only performed if it is scheduled. Blood tests should not be performed routinely and should be reserved for causes where the diagnosis is unclear from the history. For example, women who undergo a premature menopause or who have previously undergone hysterectomy may present diagnostic difficulties. In these cases, FSH > 20 IU/1 and serum oestradiol < 70 pmol/1 are diagnostic of ovarian failure. It is not necessary to perform endometrial curettage on all women prior to commencement of HRT. This

Table 4 Indications for HRT

Symptoms of oestrogen therapy
Symptoms of oestrogen dèficiency
Premature menopause
Prevention of osteoporosis
Prevention of coronary heart disease
Possible role for all women unless it is contraindicated

Table 5 Contraindications to treatment with HRT

1. Carcinoma of the breast
2. Carcinoma of the endometrium
3. Active liver disease

should be reserved for cases where there has been abnormal bleeding, which must be investigated fully before HRT is prescribed. Mammography should be performed and bone density measurement may be offered depending on local availability.

An appropriate treatment regime is prescribed and the patient is warned about common side-effects. In general, symptoms show continued improvement over the first 3 months of treatment. Review should take place 3 months after commencing treatment. Symptoms should be discussed and the patient's bleeding pattern should be considered. It has been shown that if bleeding occurs on day 10 or earlier in the progestogen phase, endometrial protection may not be satisfactory. The HRT regimen may be altered and subsequently the patient should attend for follow-up every 6 months. At these visits symptoms and bleeding patterns are reviewed and a record is made of blood pressure and weight. Breast self-examination should be taught and regular mammograms should be performed. Unscheduled vaginal bleeding must be investigated by endometrial curettage.

Benefits of hormone replacement therapy

Menopausal symptoms

Typical menopausal symptoms such as hot flushes, night sweats and insomnia are improved by HRT in the majority of women.

Osteoporosis

HRT is the treatment of choice for the prevention of postmenopausal osteoporosis. Treatment should be instituted as soon as possible after the menopause if maximal skeletal protection is to be achieved. Bone loss is halted for as long as treatment continues. Minimum bone-sparing doses of oestrogen are: conjugated equine oestrogens 0.625 mg, oestradiol valerate 2.0 mg, 17-β oestradiol (transdermal) 50 μg, oestradiol implant 50 mg. Protestins may also confer skeletal protection. Epidemiological studies suggest a 50% reduction in osteoporotic fracture incidence with 5 years of HRT use.

Cardiovascular disease

Oestrogen therapy is effective in preventing cardiovascular and cerebrovascular disease in postmenopausal women. The mechanism of this effect is through its beneficial effect on the lipid profile and in addition it may act by increasing myocardial and cerebral blood flow. Progestins do not appear to significantly impair this protection.

How long to treat?

To achieve significant protection from osteoporosis and heart disease, most practitioners would recommend a minimum duration of treatment of 5 years.

Risks of oestrogen replacement therapy

Thromboembolism

There is no clinical evidence of increased thromboembolism in patients on oestrogen replacement therapy.

Hypertension

The majority of studies report no significant change in blood pressure on continuous hormone replacement therapy.

Breast cancer

The role of HRT in the development of breast cancer remains controversial.

A meta-analysis by Steinberg et al. of 16 studies suggested an association between breast cancer and greater than 15 years' duration of oestrogen. Dupont and Page included 28 studies and suggest an increased risk of breast cancer in women taking 1.25 mg of conjugated equine oestrogens but not 0.625 mg of conjugated equine oestrogens.

Although long-term use may be associated with slightly increased breast cancer risk there is an overall decrease in mortality, and this may be due to histological confusion between hyperplasia and carcinoma in these women.

The addition of progestin does not effect the incidence of breast carcinoma and thus need not be given in hysterectomised women.

Endometrial cancer

Unopposed oestrogen therapy increases the risk of endometrial carcinoma. The addition of progestational agents has been demonstrated to reduce the incidence down to a relative index of 0.9.

ADVICE ON CONTRACEPTION AROUND THE MENOPAUSE

Although fertility around the menopause is reduced, conception can still occur. If no contraception is used around the menopause, the pregnancy rate is between 10 and 20 per 100 woman-years at age 45 and up to 5 per 100 woman-years at the age of 50. At this age pregnancy is rarely welcome and this low risk is unacceptable.

After the final menstrual period women are advised to continue contraception for 1 year if it occurs after the age of 50, and 2 years if it occurs before 50 years of age.

Combined oral contraceptives

If a woman is healthy and non-smoking there is no upper limit for combined oral contraceptive use. When does a woman change over to conventional HRT? If after discontinuing the oral contraceptive pill for 1 month and the FSH level is greater than 20 IU/1 ovarian failure is likely to have occurred. She can then use barrier forms of contraception for 1 year (i.e. 1 year post last bleed) to be certain of not conceiving.

If after stopping the combined oral contraceptive pill FSH levels are still low she is still fertile and full contraceptive precautions are needed.

Progestagen-only contraceptive

The progestagen-only pill (POP) does not suppress the rise in FSH, so FSH levels can be used to confirm the menopause. Then a similar regime as above can be followed.

Hormone replacement therapy

If the woman enters the menopause on HRT having been put on it for regulation of periods or menopausal symptoms, FSH levels will rise as with the progestagen-only pill. Therefore a similar regime can be followed. This can all be demonstrated in Table 6.

CONCLUSION

HRT is one of the great advances in preventive medicine this century. Benefits are great, side-effects are few and there are relatively few absolute contraindications.

Greater education of the public and medical world needs to take place to increase the uptake of this therapy.

Table 6 Plan for menopausal contraceptive cover

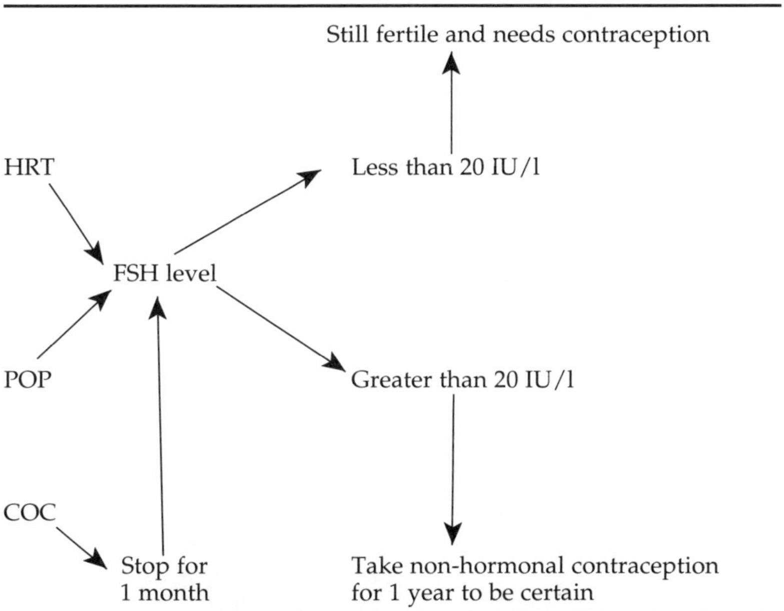

HRT = hormone replacement therapy; POP = progestagen-only pill; COC = combined oral contraceptive.

SUGGESTED READING

Buchsbaum, H. J. (ed.) (1983). *The Menopause: Clinical Perspectives in Obstetrics and Gynaecology.* Springer-Verlag, New York.

Drife, J. O. and Studd, J. W. W. (eds) (1990). *HRT and Osteoporosis.* Based on the 22nd Study Group of the Royal College of Obstetricians and Gynaecologists. Springer-Verlag, London.

Dupont, W. D. and Page, D. L. (1991). Menopausal oestrogen replacement therapy and breast cancer. *Arch. Intern. Med.*, **151**, 67–72.

Session, D., Kelly, A. and Jewelewicz, R. (1993). Current concepts of oestrogen replacement therapy in the menopause. *Fertil. Steril.*, **59**, 277–284.

Steinberg, K. K., Thacker, S. B., Smith, J., Stroup, D. F., Zack, M. M. and Flanders, W. D. (1991). A meta analysis of the effects of oestrogen replacement therapy on the risk of breast cancer. *JAMA*, **265**, 1985–1990.

Studd, J. W. W. and Whitehead, M. I. (eds) (1988). *The Menopause.* Blackwell Scientific, Oxford.

Index

Index compiled by Liza Weinkove